Management Issues
for a
DERMATOLOGIST

Management Issues for a DERMATOLOGIST

Editors

S Sacchidanand
Registrar (Evaluation)
Rajiv Gandhi University of Health Sciences
Bengaluru, India
President, Indian Association of Dermatologists,
Venereologists and Leprologists (IADVL)

Formerly
Professor and HOD
Department of Dermatology
BMC and RI
Bengaluru, India

Bhanu Prakash
Associate Professor
Department of Dermatology
Vydehi Hospital, Bengaluru, India

Foreword
SDN Guptha

JAYPEE BROTHERS MEDICAL PUBLISHERS (P) LTD

New Delhi • Ahmedabad • Bengaluru • Chennai • Hyderabad • Kochi
Kolkata • Lucknow • Mumbai • Nagpur • St Louis (USA)

Published by

Jitendar P Vij
Jaypee Brothers Medical Publishers (P) Ltd

Corporate Office
4838/24 Ansari Road, Daryaganj, **New Delhi** - 110 002, India, +91-11-43574357 (30 lines)

Registered Office
B-3 EMCA House, 23/23B Ansari Road, Daryaganj, **New Delhi** 110 002, India
Phones: +91-11-23272143, +91-11-23272703, +91-11-23282021,
+91-11-23245672, Rel: +91-11-32558559 Fax: +91-11-23276490, +91-11-23245683
e-mail: jaypee@jaypeebrothers.com, Website: www.jaypeebrothers.com

Branches

- 2/B, Akruti Society, Jodhpur Gam Road Satellite
  Ahmedabad 380 015 Phones: +91-79-26926233, Rel: +91-79-32988717
  Fax: +91-79-26927094 e-mail: ahmedabad@jaypeebrothers.com
- 202 Batavia Chambers, 8 Kumara Krupa Road, Kumara Park East
  Bengaluru 560 001 Phones: +91-80-22285971, +91-80-22382956, +91-80-22372664
  Rel: +91-80-32714073, Fax: +91-80-22281761 e-mail: bangalore@jaypeebrothers.com
- 282 IIIrd Floor, Khaleel Shirazi Estate, Fountain Plaza, Pantheon Road
  Chennai 600 008 Phones: +91-44-28193265, +91-44-28194897,
  Rel: +91-44-32972089 Fax: +91-44-28193231 e-mail: chennai@jaypeebrothers.com
- 4-2-1067/1-3, 1st Floor, Balaji Building, Ramkote Cross Road
  Hyderabad 500 095 Phones: +91-40-66610020, +91-40-24758498, Rel:+91-40-32940929
  Fax:+91-40-24758499 e-mail: hyderabad@jaypeebrothers.com
- No. 41/3098, B & B1, Kuruvi Building, St. Vincent Road
  Kochi 682 018, Kerala Phones: +91-484-4036109, +91-484-2395739, +91-484-2395740
  e-mail: kochi@jaypeebrothers.com
- 1-A Indian Mirror Street, Wellington Square
  Kolkata 700 013 Phones: +91-33-22651926, +91-33-22276404, +91-33-22276415
  Rel: +91-33-32901926, Fax: +91-33-22656075, e-mail: kolkata@jaypeebrothers.com
- Lekhraj Market III, B-2, Sector-4, Faizabad Road, Indira Nagar
  Lucknow 226 016 Phones: +91-522-3040553, +91-522-3040554
  e-mail: lucknow@jaypeebrothers.com
- 106 Amit Industrial Estate, 61 Dr SS Rao Road, Near MGM Hospital, Parel
  Mumbai 400012 Phones: +91-22-24124863, +91-22-24104532, Rel: +91-22-32926896
  Fax: +91-22-24160828 e-mail: mumbai@jaypeebrothers.com
- "KAMALPUSHPA" 38, Reshimbag, Opp. Mohota Science College, Umred Road
  Nagpur 440 009 (MS) Phone: Rel: +91-712-3245220,
  Fax: +91-712-2704275 e-mail: nagpur@jaypeebrothers.com

USA Office
1745, Pheasant Run Drive, Maryland Heights (Missouri), MO 63043, USA, Ph: 001-636-6279734
e-mail: jaypee@jaypeebrothers.com, anjulav@jaypeebrothers.com

Management Issues for a Dermatologist

First Edition: **2009**

Reprint: 2024

ISBN 978-81-8448-594-3

Typeset at JPBMP typesetting unit
Printed in India

Contributors

DS Krupashankar
Consultant Dermatologist
Manipal Hospital
Bengaluru, India
dermakrupa@yahoo.com

HM Omprakash
Consultant Dermatologist
Vikram Hospital
Mysore, India
drhmomprakash@yahoo.com

SC Rajendran
Professor of Dermatology
Vydehi Hospital
Bengaluru, India
Dr_rajendran080@yahoo.co.in

N Vishwanathan
Chartered Accountant
vishy1962@yahoo.com

S Ravidatha
Cost Accountant
ravidatha@rediffmail.com

GN Subbanna
gnsubbanna@yahoo.co.in

KH Satyanarayana Rao
Consultant Dermatologist,
Central Government Health Services
konanurrao@gmail.com

Gurcharan Singh
Professor and HOD
Department of Dermatology
Sri Devaraj Urs Medical College
Kolar, India
gsdrsingh@gmail.com

AL Shyam Prasad
Professor of Dermatology
MS Ramaiah Teaching Hospital
Bengaluru, India
Prashyam2@yahoo.co.in

Bhanu Prakash
Associate Professor
Department of Dermatology
Vydehi Hospital
Bengaluru, India
drbhanuprakash@rediffmail.com

GR Kanthraj
Department of Dermatology
JSS Hospital
Mysore, India
kanthacad@yahoo.com.

Mysore Venkat Ram
Consultant Dermatologist
Venkat Charmalaya
Bengaluru, India
mysorevenkat@hotmail.com

S Sacchidanand
Registrar (Evaluation)
Rajiv Gandhi University of Health Sciences
Bengaluru, India
President, IADVL
sacchi1260@gmail.com

Foreword

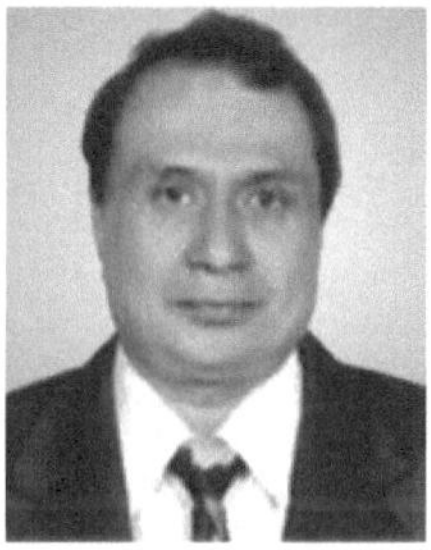

Recent years have witnessed an explosion of knowledge among the common man leading to increased awareness of issues like consumer activity, legal issues and social rights. In the last decade or so there has been an ongoing effort to incorporate management issues in almost all forms of work fields. We doctors cannot afford to be left behind. With the changing scenario in health sector where corporatisation and third party payers are ruling the hospitals, we will be risking ourselves if we do not fall in line with these issues.

Similarly, we have also noticed an exponential increase in the activity and advance happening to this 'poor cousin of medicine' i.e. Dermatology. Dermatology has moved away from being a one man army department to a superspecialty department. Therefore, it has become imperative that we as doctors in general and dermatologists in particular, are aware of these issues and be prepared to encounter any problems arising out of these in our day-to-day practice whether we are sitting in our clinic or in a department of any teaching/research institution.

While going through the book, I was surprised at the numerous issues which have been brought out. I request all my fellow colleagues to read and understand these issues. Do not allow a consumer court or a government agency to send us a notice in our clinic and then spend more time to running around from pillar to post to sort out these issues. Rather understand and incorporate some of the wise ideas given in this book and stay away from troubled waters.

When Dr S Sacchidanand asked me to write a foreword to this book, I was wondering whether a book of this nature was required for a dermatologist. But after having read this book, I am left with no option but to be convinced to say that it is a must. I congratulate him and his team for having worked on this idea. I am sure this book will be a treasure for all dermatologists—students and teachers, young and old dermatologists alike.

SDN Guptha
MD, DVD
Senior Consultant Dermatologist
Sri Sathya Sai Hospital, Bengaluru

Preface

Having done specialization in Dermatology, we always aspire for achieving higher ends as excellent professionals. As we embrace Dermatology, we also invariably have to embrace the other face of our life-management. Yet unlike all other professionals in various fields who are exposed to certain management juggernauts from the day they begin their careers, we are almost totally unaware of it. With the globalization at its peak today, there are many issues which have begun to affect us almost every second in our practice. Issues like waste management, medicolegal issues, drug trial issues, computers, etc. though very important, have still remained a gray area to many of us. Added to these new issues, are the already existing problems of not having understood our old foes: our financial needs, pricing or how to handle our patients and our staff.

This book is an effort in that direction to make the people realize the existence of such issues. It gives a brief profile of these issues and helps understand the various non-dermatological mysteries one has to encounter.

Though it was tempting to touch upon many other issues, we have purposely kept it confined to certain burning issues only. We, with your support and positive response, look forward to widening the scope of the book in the future days.

The book has been authored by dermatologists who have a wide array of experience and knowledge in the topics which they have covered. Also some topics which are clearly out of a dermatologist's domain have been authored by specialists in those particular fields. I do hope that each author's unique style of writing will stimulate us to think and act upon these issues.

Dr S Sacchidanand, the "Management Legend in Dermatology" took the initiative by dreaming about this book. He then put this into action by asking us to work on this project. We thank him for having posed faith in us by asking to coordinate this project. We do hope we have not let him down.

We thank all the authors for having contributed by writing the topics asked for and having done it in time. As coordinators, we look forward to all the readers to send in their feedback to help us learn and understand more. We firmly believe that we dermatologists must perceive ourselves as members of a professional community whose collective strength can only enhance each of its individual members.

S Sacchidanand
Bhanu Prakash

Contents

Career Options for a Dermatologist

DS Krupashankar
Consultant Dermatologist
Manipal Hospital, Bangalore
dermakrupa@yahoo.com

1

INTRODUCTION

Dermatology is practiced by Dermatologists; the fate of one is that of the other.

No more semantics or pontificating. There is an exchange of cash and respect between doctors and patients. A large number of people want to cash in on this action. These characters will be collectively referred to as interlopers.

Their role is apparently to facilitate medical care to patients. Interlopers do not work for free. They interrupt the supply chain between doctors and patients and hijack the transactions.

This results in higher costs to patients and lower respect to doctors and Lower remuneration to doctors. Over time interlopers marginalize the primary stake holders, in medical care, namely the patients and doctors in their relentless pursuit of efficient profiteering.

Interlopers include:

- Health insurance companies
- Third party payers
- Managed health care
- Corporate hospital administrators
- Branded chain clinics

Insurance companies make a profit of around 20%. For every Rs 10 you pay, you can get a maximum of Rs 8. Insurance operates on rejections and exclusions.

Insurance does not cover ambulatory care. The person who sells the policy and the one who settles the claims are different. Insurance companies employ doctors to scrutinize claims to assist rejection. They employ third parties to streamline collections, aid rejections and deny payments to medical institutions.

They strike deals directly with HR managers of companies and eat into your pay packet and cut off the direct disbursement of health care costs available hitherto. They do not support or fund research, not even outcome studies.

WHAT TO TELL PATIENTS

They must lobby in the following directions:

- Insist that there will be no third party administrators involved in insurance disbursement, this is already happening in vehicle insurance
- Demand bonus or reduction in premium for every year of non-claim or denied claim

- Insist that the policy seller be the disburser
- Lobby for a law against imposition of health insurance from a single vendor on all employees by the employer or the company's HR department.
- Do not buy health insurance, instead put money in a recurring deposit or open ended mutual fund and use it for medical expenses when needed
- Buy shares of a health insurance company
- Here are some excerpts from my hand out to patients who insist that their insurer will cover the services I have to offer.

  In my experience, admission for skin diseases entails hospitalization charges in addition to the regular expenses, followed by many trips to the insurance office ending in a rejection on technical grounds.
- At this point, your agent will ask you to request your doctor to do the paperwork for a disease that **is** covered under insurance, in other words he encourages you to involve yourself and your treating physician in insurance fraud
- When you put forth this seemingly innocent idea to your doctor, your angered physician will ask you to go climb a tree
- You feel humiliated and now believe that the doctor who saved your life is an obstructionist and a heartless enemy
- When you buy health insurance, you spend money to lose freedom, suffer deception and a long and tormenting sense of denied entitlement that is deleterious to mental health.

CORPORATE HOSPITALS

These are 200 to 800 bedded hospitals covering all specialties, with emphasis on those specialties currently considered most profitable and peopled with super specialists, i.e. people with 3 degrees such as DM; Mch etc. Dermatology is included in these institutions generally as a fire engine service, i.e. something that has to be there for completions sake. The owners or their representatives have a very poor or skewed idea of what dermatology involves, but has a vague understanding that something is happening, but not enough to involve themselves in a study of the ground realities and possibilities, and certainly not enough to make heavy investments. This is a window of opportunity.

CORPORATE MINI HOSPITALS

These are 100 to 200 bedded hospitals with ICU and emergency care and aim at neutralizing the nursing home business and are generally dotted on the peripheries of an expanding city, the erstwhile catchment areas of the superspeciality hospitals. Dermatology may or may not find a place here. The approach is similar to that of individual nursing home owners who classify dermatologists as laid back characters who spend time attending to trivial problems. This is a window of opportunity.

CORPORATE HOSPITAL CLINICS

Aim at neutralizing the polyclinics and have a pharmacy, diagnostic center, Ambulance service to the parent superspeciality hospital and facilities for consultants on time slots and an agreement to feed the parent institution with admissions by the consultants. Dermatologists do have an opening here, but may be obliged to spend all their time motoring from slot to slot and land up spending on road, time better spent with a patient or books and journals.

- Are all these not a wonderful opportunity for just qualified Dermatologists and junior Dermatologists?
- What is wrong in joining these?

One can always learn and move on into ones practice with the benefit of the institutions name, and divert a few patients as well. Not really, because:

- Institutions will get your best hours and your best years
- Institutions get herded patients who are increasingly brand loyal.
- Your services receive a fraction of their market worth, with the remaining raked in by the health care delivery system peopled with busybodies from diverse backgrounds, including occasionally from clinical medicine.
- You get paid peanuts
- If you pay peanuts, you get monkeys
- You run the risk of becoming a monkey.
- The powers that be speak with great ambition, but dig their heels into the ground and become obstinate as mules when it comes to making investments in dermatology, you will spend considerable time and energy trying to get a level of basic care that the pampered specialties get easily. Besides whenever you ask for anything, you are given the impression of being a beggar or supplicant, and an impression is conveyed of a favor being granted to you when you put in place what the patients need.

Corporate hospital strategies include:

- Visibility
- Hours
- Ambience
- Access and facility
- Full timers
- Market watching
- Marketing
- Damming the catchments

Visibility

Why do we need it?

We need it because of the Geographical fixity of doctor vs. the mobility of the earning population. Most jobs today involve relocation, travel and on site stays.

The paying population will not be around for you to build a word of mouth reputation. You need to be a noisy colorful bird of the jungle to be seen and sought.

Role of Associations in Visibility

Most professional associations have large funds sitting around unutilized. A few strategies can be thought of to utilize it for the benefit of the members.

Advertise the website on hoardings, vehicles and individual vehicles of members as well as in other visible and audible media.

Hire full time webmaster for regular upgrading. Remunerate the concerned office bearer who will work for the benefit of the rest.

Promote the organizations and their members to consumer groups directly.

Create a coca cola like icon and empower individual dermatologists with it.

Ready members to handle the result of campaigns by a 3 part strategy targeting individual common diseases.

For example, run 4 weekend courses on the consensus management of acne including approach, work-up, prescription and follow-up in February.

Flood the media with the message, the means to identify and access dermatologists in their local area in March and collect and analyze the output of efforts in April to refine the plan for that disease for the next year. 4 to six campaigns can be run per annum. This will standardize care, guide patients to the people best qualified to treat them and eliminate one-upmanship.

Protocols and guidelines have to be in place for the 20 commonest diseases we treat in order to eliminate the yawning differences we see in the level of care offered by different practitioners for the same disease.

Permit practices and individual doctors to upload their links and pay a rent to the associations website if they wish to give more information than the standard format provided by the website.

Hours

Corporate hospitals provide consultant services from 7.30 am to 8.30 pm Monday to Saturday Plus 9 am to 5 pm on Sunday, totaling to 86 patient accessible hours.

A Stand alone dermatologist working full time can provide only 48 to 56 Patient hours in a week if working out of a single location and less if in more places as time is lost in transit.

However, 2 dermatologists can deliver 96 quality hours, 3 can do more 2 minds are better than 1 and 6 hands can do a lot more than 2, it makes sense for 2 or more people to share the same infrastructure and increase patient convenience.

Ambience

Ambience is constituted of the following physical factors:

- Temperature, i.e. cooling, heating, ventilation air conditioning costs.
- Sights, i.e. décor
- Smell, i.e. general hygiene ventilation and personal hygiene of personnel
- Physical comfort, i.e. furnishing, space and lines of movement for people.
- Human interaction implies the presence, pleasant nature and facilitatory approach of all personnel other than the doctor.
- Ambience costs money
- A shared facility makes this possible and affordable
- 1 secretary, 1 cleaner, 1 airconditioner, 1 nurse, 1 genset versus 4 of each if 4 such people decide to practice together.

Non-medical Administrators

Practice sycophancy and expect the same, mistake it for loyalty, are intolerant of a difference of opinion, and cannot understand the reasons behind certain disagreements from doctors on account of being ignorant of medical knowledge as well as the patient management paradigm.

Easily influenced by slogans, titles, days, celebrations.

Insecure for being in the midst of a lot of intelligent people and having to manage them.

Intolerant and Afraid of True Competence

Highly resentful of the praise, reverence, respect that patients and the general population give to doctors and feel personally offended and small in the presence of a medical luminary.

They resent the easy camaraderie and communication between doctors of different specialties and seniority, never having been exposed to the collegial spirit that creates a sense of fraternity among professionals in their years of training.

Predatory in their approach to individual doctors and smaller medical establishments. I have personally heard them refer to a doctor as "that fellow" and other choice unprintable expletives. Their board room talk is peppered with lines such as " neutralize that doctor", teach this bu***r a lesson","kill that nursing home", "swallow up this hospital" "finish off that consultant", all this sounds rather strange coming from people who claim to be in the life saving business.

Chain gangs or branded clinic chains are a good place to learn the value the general public places on enhancement services as offered by cosmetic dermatology, but spending too much time there has its hazards. Such as:

Practice on the Edge of Quackery

Application of unproven or low evidence technologies and techniques.

Dangers of incentives to doctors for promoting procedures carried out in their absence by technicians.

This leads to unclear post counseling course of those who undergo the above procedures, leading to erosion of rational thinking by the dermatologist and the risks of a low, manipulative remuneration.

Remember that if you feed Homo sapiens enough peanuts, he will turn into a monkey.

Rheumatologists are a great help in managing many of our patients with multisystemic disease, but because of corporate marketing, they will receive patients with collagen vascular diseases, skin diseases with joint manifestations.

All multisystem diseases with skin manifestations, anything that seems mysterious to a physician or general practitioner often leading to a delay in diagnosis and needless expenditure for the patient.

Immunologists deal with any disease where the word or concept "immune" is involved. I have encountered patients treated with the following disorders by immunologists: Chronic actinic dermatitis, Alopecia areata, Urticaria, Delayed pressure urticaria, Impetigo contagiosa, Lichen planus, AIDS.

Internists are a lot more cautious in their management of skin disorders now as compared to a few years ago and do not attempt to cure all with topical steroids or steroid antimicrobial combinations, however, make sure if the word skin is involved, you are involved , which is not too difficult in these litigious times and make them your partners in in-patient management.

Many of us are drawn to institutions for the traditional institutional advantages.

Such as a library with access to texts, journals, monographs, Record keeping, clinical meetings, interaction with other specialties, Nomenclature/designation.

Fraternity and teaching-learning and most importantly access to expensive infrastructure and equipment.

With the changing times the Institutional advantages are in doubt.

Library: any 2 standard texts of dermatology is adequate for regular practice as well as diagnosis and management of rare disorders.

Abstracts of most leading journals are available online and many journals including the IJDVL are available full text online. Journals are in any case browsed and full text read only when directly relevant to ones work or a given patient with a rare manifestation or rare disease.

Monographs are delivered by pharma companies in quantities more than you can read Record keeping on the computer, or better a laptop is superior to the paper based systems of hospitals. Clinical meetings of your local derma community are another source of effortless learning as is that of the other specialists if you were to identify a good local IMA branch. Nomenclature/designation can be as you please if you own your own firm. The needs of Fraternity and Teaching-learning are met by the over 5 conferences per annum at various levels of your specialty.

Access to expensive equipment is no longer an insurmountable obstacle as in the past on account of the following developments:

- Declining equipment cost
- Smaller lighter portable equipment

- Indigenization
- Easy loans
- Very low cost techniques with comparable results
- There are many dermatologists who share equipment on predetermined days of a week or a month or place it in one area and access at will.
- Lease and day hiring are other options.

In the foreseeable future, the Institution bound specialties will be

- Anesthesia
- Intensive care
- Neurosurgery
- Cardiac surgery

The advent of Dermatologic Subspecialties such as Pediatric dermatology. Dermatologic surgery, Dermatopathology, Cosmetic dermatology, Trichology is an opportunity to spend more time to learn a small area well and works well in set ups with a comfortable salary, or where the basic fee per service is rewarding. We need to know whether in a resource poor developing country, we can afford to have more and more people doing less and less and indulge in longer years of training. Salary paying employers, patients, third party payers and the doctors in training themselves will demand value for money and value for time. The long years in training and the shrinking private practice prospects and the uncertain corporate hospital machinations is already driving many young bright minds away from medicine as an option.

Advancement in technology will benefit the individual said Alvin Toffler and you have witnessed the opportunity revolution unleashed by the mobile phone.

The world's most efficient, successful and competent organizations have around 20 people said Alvin Toffler. To us this may mean that being in a big behemoth organization with 2500 people in a glass and chrome edifice may not be the key to, or even an ingredient of success.

The morphologists skills are unique and are had only by Dermatologists, Pathologists, and Dermatopathologists.

This can result only from supervised training and cannot be acquired by any one else or any other means, putting us in a position of relative advantage.

Everything that can be digitized will be digitized said-Thomas Freidman, author of "The world is flat". This means that all the medical knowledge will be available to any one who wants it and a dermatologist can hone his skills in the prescription writing of any branch. The day is not far away when you can treat the systemic manifestations of a disease with skin signs.

If you compile 1 smart idea on your computer once, you can use it an endless number of times.

Memory is the foundation of intelligence.

World class memory is available for less than Rs 25000.

Here are some medical management protocols.
'What will you do with a patient who has subcorneal pustular dermatosis?
Serum G6PDH assay to consider dapsone therapy and
Serum protein electrophoresis
Serum immunoelectrophoresis
Urinalysis
Urine for Bence Jones proteins to rule out the common associations.

A Dapsone protocol could include:
- G6PDH, CBC before therapy and 1 month later
- CBC, SGPT, Methemoglobin keeping in mind the common problems with dapsone.
- Any dermatologist can prepare such digital documents for use and for sharing with colleagues.
- All things being equal what distinguishes the leading organization is **culture** says Edward de bono doctor, physiologist, psychologist and inventor of the concept of lateral thinking.

Culture problems among dermatologists and doctors in general are assumptions such as:
- Suffering is a virtue
- Poverty is a virtue
- Talking and thinking of money is a sin
- All patients need and deserve free treatment and it is my personal responsibility to provide it to them
- What will my patients think if they find out I have heard of money?
- Medicine is a noble profession
- Poverty ennobles
- If I remain poor I will be noble

"Poverty does not ennoble, it only makes one mean and wretched"
—Somerset Maugham

And then we have more culture problems:

- I need to prove that I am the smartest doctor in the world
- To do this I need to prove everyone else a fool
- Inability to share respect
- Inability to trust
- Inability and unwillingness to share money
- Deadly envy
- Resentment of others' success.

This leads to the need for fancy nomenclature which stems from the desire to appear smarter and more distinguished than others:

- Cosmetologist
- Dermatosurgeon
- Aesthetic surgeon
- Cosmetic surgeon
- Allergy specialist
- Immunologist
- Trichologist

What is wrong with dermatologist? After all most of our patients are just beginning to use that word.

Strategies for the future for senior dermatologists:

- Hire juniors
- Increase hours and offer partnership
- Increase earnings
- Increase services
- Increase revenue streams
- Compile skills, standards and protocols
- Grow, grow, grow and enjoy your growth.

Strategies for the future for junior dermatologists:

- Get together
- Do not compete with each other across the street and sink collectively
- Pool resources into a good basic infrastructure
- Get a senior of standing to collaborate with you
- Organize around a sound and dependable system of incorporation
- Prepare for long and inconvenient hours
- Lone rangers are for comic books
- Understand that we are all different from each other and this is an advantage
- Laugh all the way to the bank

2

Designing a Dermatology Center

HM Omprakash
Consultant Dermatologist
Vikram Hospital, Mysore
drhmomprakash@yahoo.com

INTRODUCTION

Dermatology in a past few decades has grown exponentially. To master nearly 2,000 diseases[1] in a short 2 to 3 years of postgraduation time is a herculean task. One glaring omission we find in our curriculum is how does one manage his or her practice?

The planning of dermatology practice starts from the days of medical college. One has to make up one's mind whether he is going into private practice which is financially fertile or institutional/medical college practice which is professionally fertile with a fixed income or a few exceptions wherein one can have both institute practice and private practice. Next important decision is where one's heart and mind fits – i.e. subspecialty. Just a look at the scope for growth would certainly surprise everyone.

1. General dermatology
2. Dermatopathology
3. Pediatric dermatology
4. Procedural dermatology
5. Medical dermatology
6. Hospital dermatology (hospitalists)
7. Cosmetic dermatology
8. Laboratory research
9. Dermatologic epidemiology[2]

"One of the most common misconceptions I see among recently graduated residents is the focus they place on the cosmetic side while ignoring the medical side of dermatology"—these are the words of Dr. Joel Schlessinger.[3] How very right. It is the general dermatology consultation which feeds cases to cosmetic dermatology.

Having specialized the next big step for a dermatologist is getting started. This requires careful planning with regards to two aspects

1. Manpower
2. Material

MANPOWER

Whether a medical college or private practice the very backbone of a department is the manpower.

This includes:

(a) Front office staff (b) Dermatologists (c) Nursing staff/Nursing aids (d) Housekeeping staff (e) Security personnel (f) helping hand.

a. Front office staff: The front office people need not have any special educational qualification. All that is required here is– people's people. The staff should have patience and make the clients visit comfortable. In many practice the front office manages the phone, billing and scheduling appointments. But in a busy practice the phone and billing can be separated.

b. Dermatologists: In a group practice it is very important to have likeminded colleagues pooling their talent and finance to a common end. A general dermatologist and a procedurally inclined dermatologist could be an ideal combination. But a team could easily be poisoned, if there is lack of communication and common goals. So before teaming, employing–wait. Better be safe than sorry. Also look into the option of a visiting-plastic and reconstructive surgeon and anesthetist.

c. Nursing staff/nursing aids: In a general dermatology outpatient practice a nursing aid with basics of asepsis is that all required. But if one does lot of procedural dermatology a single nursing staff to supervise- sterilization, disinfection and operation theater assistance will do. Also if one has a phototherapy unit functioning, a trained phototherapist can run the chamber even outside office hours to help the working clients to access the facility at their hour of choice.

But when hiring a nurse/aid or other personnel, remember the golden rule of human relations-

"Take your time; it is better to find the right person slowly than the wrong person fast".

Also don't allow bad staff to linger long, for they could have a bad influence on the rest. Also have a policy manual of (1) daily duty hours (2) leave policy (3) work schedule (4) list of procedures performed and the role of the staff in each procedure (5) sterilization and disinfection (6) housekeeping protocol-be it bath room or consultation room or waiting lobby (7) biopsy and laboratory sample handling, labeling and filing the reports (8) consent for surgery (9) OT register, phototherapy register (10) medical case record filing and retrieval (11) stock inventory.

d, e, f. Housekeeping, security and helping hand personnel should also have a work schedule written and they should adhere to, be it switching the generator, operating a lift, handling biopsy specimens or blood samples or daily cleanliness of the premises. In fact they form the hidden backbone of one's practice, and often ignored.

MATERIAL

The material investment in the form of building and instruments forms the next important decision one has to make.

Building Infrastructure

In private practice the floor space requirement depends upon whether it is solo or group practice. According to Lea Chantam, a health care writer this could vary from 1,350 square feet to 3,000 square feet. This takes into account

1. Waiting lobby
2. Reception
3. Consultation room
4. Examination room
5. Procedure room.

But in a major city this could be expensive proposition and majority of us settle for less than 1,000 square feet. By scheduling the appointments telephonically one can practice comfortable in a lesser space – for example

Waiting lobby	Reception	Consultation-1	Phototherapy	Operation theater	Total
64 square feet	32 square feet	100 square feet	100 square feet	144 square feet	440 square feet.
5.76 square meter	3.24 square meter	9 square meter	9 square meter	12 square meter	39 square meter

But if one looks at the medical council of India guidelines, one is in for a surprise with regards to a medical college set up.

Prof. and HOD/Sr. consultant	1 room	18 sq.m.
Assoc Prof/Consultants	2 rooms	15 sq.m. each
Asst Prof/Jr. consultants(3)	1 room	20 sq. m.
Tutors/residents	1 room	15 sq.m.
Department office cum clerical room		12 sq.m.
Working accommodation for nonteaching staff		12 sq.m.

- Regarding the operation theater floor space that are recommended ranges from-
  10 × 10 feet[4]
  12 × 12 feet[5]
  12 × 15 feet[6]

However, the IADVL national guidelines taskforce is considering recommending a minimum size of dermatosurgery theater to be 12 × 12 feet, in India. This is based on the fact that the center stage of the theater is the operating table occupying at least 6 feet in length. In the eventuality of the surgeon having to resuscitate the patient, additional 3 feet is required at the head end. The same applies to the foot end. So the length of the theater should be minimum 12 feet. The breadth may be 12 feet.[7]

Also one has to bear in mind the financial implications of every square foot. In a city like Bangalore the rental per square foot could be anywhere between Rupees 100, to a minimum of 30 rupees.

Apart from space other factors like-lighting, electrical plug points, instruments, operation tables, chairs, sterilization and disinfection equipments, biomedical waste management, water supply, bathrooms, electricity backup issues have to be addressed. This can be got from the IADVL national guidelines for setting up a operation theater.[7]

The basic consultation room requirements are:

1. Work desk
2. Chairs for patients and consultant
3. Examination table
4. Loupe
5. Wood's lamp
6. Compound microscope
7. Various stains—Gram, Zeil Nielson and KOH 10%
8. Desktop personal computer/Laptop
9. Digital camera-3 megapixel
10. Weighing machine
11. Mercury manometer
12. Stethoscope
13. Reference textbooks.

However, one can add-dermatoscope, imaging software, trichogram software.

With regards to other equipment—Cryosurgery unit, Dewar tank, Radiosurgery unit and phototherapy unit could be basic. But budget constraints and local needs of patients has to be taken into consideration. These devices are locally manufactured and some are be imported. But one has to weigh the cost, safety of device, backup service and certification by governing bodies like-ISI, CE and USFDA.

Lasers for scar correction, hair reduction could be ideal for beginners. Vascular and pigment specific laser requires sufficient work load to maintain the device, hence may be optional. Hiring these devices could also be an option.

The patient data could be stored in the conventional paper folders. However, electronic medical records could be looked into. Before buying this software one should see the reputation of the vendor, the service he offers in case of breakdown and backup of data.

Lastly every patient is a potential litigant. Hence taking professional indemnity insurance is a must.

To conclude, starting once practice either at medical college or private practice requires careful planning. All said and done, apart from – Man-power and Material, one does require grandfatherly advice. So one should read and reread Dr Lawrence M Field's-"(Great) Grandfatherly advice for Young(er) dermatologic surgeon.[8]

Acknowledgement of scientific inputs: Dr S.C. Rajendran MD, DVD former professor and Head, Department of Dermatology, St John's Medical College, Bangalore. Dr Jayadev Betkerur, MD, DVD, Professor and head Department of Dermatology, JSS Medical College, Mysore. Dr kantharaj G.R. MD, Assistant Professor of Dermatology, JSS Medical College, Mysore. Dr Bhanuprakash, Assistant Professor of Dermatology, Videyi Institute of Medical Sciences, Bangalore.

REFERENCES

1. The dermatologist's work – in – chapter one-Introduction and historical bibliography; In RH Champion, JL Burton, DA Burns, SM Breathnach (Eds): Rook's Textbook of Dermatology, 6th edition, 1998, Blackwell scientific, oxford, England.
2. Paul R Bergstresser. Sub specialization in Dermatology: 03 Apr 07, www.dermaquest.com. Last viewed on 8-12-2008.
3. Joel Schlesinger, Starting or transitioning into cosmetic dermatology July 2007, www.dermaquest.com. Last viewed on 8-12-2008
4. Satish S Savant, Deepak Gore. Instruments, equipment and universal precautions, In Satish S Savant (Eds): Textbook of Dermatosurgery and Cosmetology; Mumbai, India, published by Association of Scientific cosmetologists and dermatosurgeons, 2005;26-34.
5. Clifford Lawrence: Chapter2- Equipment, in Clifford Lawrence: An introduction to dermatological surgery; London. Published by Churchill Livingstone, 2002;5.
6. Walter P Unger. 22. B. The surgical suite, in Walter P Unger, Ronald Shapiro: Hair Transplantation; New York, Marcel dekker, 2004;833-34.
7. IADVL national guidelines-"Minimum standard guidelines of care on requirements for setting up a dermatosurgery theater" (in press).
8. Lawrence M Field—"(Great) Grandfatherly advice for Young(er) dermatologic surgeon", Journal of cutaneous and aesthetic surgery, Jul-Dec 2008; Vol-1, Issue-2, 106-07.

3

Financial Considerations for Starting a Dermatology Center

SC Rajendran
Professor of Dermatology
Vydehi Hospital, Bangalore
Dr_rajendran080@yahoo.co.in

Plan your practice as a dermatologist or dermatosurgeon or aesthetic practice. Presently it is better to practice clinical dermatology as the priority and practice dermatosurgery and aesthetic practice as a secondary practice. The reason for this in today's practice in India is lot of entrepreneurs are involved in dermatology practice, for example, Skin care, hair care, hair removal, body shaping, under eye bag's treatment, fillers, botillium toxin (soft tissue augmentation). These facilities can be advertised, give incentives, requires different market promotions. As a dermatologist, it is difficult to compete with such entrepreneurs so we should have a common understanding among our close professional colleagues before starting our practice.

BUSINESS PLAN

Develop a Business Plan

- Discuss the ownership of the business and the legal structure
- List the skills and experience which you posses to introduce as services
- Highlight your special cares. For example, For vitiligo, following treatment modalities are provided:
  - Phototherapy, UVA, NB-UVB
  - Targeted phototherapy
  - Vitiligo surgeries
  - Vitiligo culture suspension etc.
- Discuss the advantages you and your business have over your competitors
- Identify the customer demand for your product/service
- Decide on the pricing strategy.

Financial considerations to be kept in mind when starting out:

- Loan applications
- Capital equipment and supply list
- Balance sheet
- Breakeven analysis
- Proforma income projections (profit and loss statements)
- Three-year summary
- Detail by month, first year
- Detail by quarters, second and third years
- Assumptions upon which projections were based
- Proforma cash flow.

Involve an auditor to take a professional advice.

Businesses have assets and so they could not, even if they wanted to, immediately turn these into cash at the end of each period. Real businesses also owe money to suppliers and to tax authorities, and the proprietors do not withdraw all their original capital and profits at the end of each period. Businesses also have liabilities.

Deliberate on these issues before starting out on new ventures:

- How good are you at making decisions? Small business owners are required to make decisions constantly - often quickly, independently, and under pressure.
- Do you have the physical and emotional stamina to run a business? Can you face six or seven 12-hour work days every week?
- How well do you plan and organize? Research indicates that poor planning is responsible for most business failures. Good organization of financials, inventory, schedules, and production can help you avoid many pitfalls.
- Plan your clinic and home nearby so that your travel time in busy metros can be avoided. By this you will be saving time and your fuel expenditure, driver expenditure, etc. You can allocate this budget for good marketing.
- How will the business affect your family? The first few years of business start up can be hard on family life. It is important for family members to know what to expect and for you to be able to trust that they will support you during this time. There also may be financial difficulties until the business becomes profitable, which could take months or years. You may have to adjust to a lower standard of living or put family assets at risk in the short-term.

FINANCIAL CONSIDERATIONS

- Explain your source and the amount of initial equity capital.
- Develop a monthly operating budget for the first year.
- Develop an expected return on investment and monthly cash flow for the first year.
- Provide projected income statements and balance sheets for a two-year period.

Take help of an auditor to look after the accounts.

Initially depending on your capability start your clinic at three levels.

LEVEL 1: Provide basic dermatology care like consultations and small procedures.

a. Space required: Waiting room of 10 × 15 ft, Consultation room of 8 × 8 ft, Procedure room 8 × 8 ft, Toilet 5 × 6 ft, Total space required around 300 sq ft. Rental of 300 × 30 = 9000/- Rs + your initial deposit depends on the place.
b. Capital expenditure should be your furniture's, interiors, air condition etc. should be between Rs. 20000/- to 30000/-
c. Equipments: Simple equipments like electrocoquetry, cryo equipments and other minor instruments. should be between Rs. 50000/- to 100000/-

Level 1 clinic should not go beyond 500000 for all your capital investments.

LEVEL 2: Should be between 500000/- to 150000 lakhs

a. Space required: Around 600 to 800 sq ft.
b. Capital expenditure should be 500000/- to 100000/- for equipments.
c. At this point one should always think about sharing part of this equipment budget with another colleague, so that you can use the equipment as and when required.
d. Always analyze when people buy equipments with your colleagues, and not by the person or the company from whom you are buying the equipment.
e. Suppose you want to buy a laser or a light source share with your colleague, 50% of your capital expenditure towards the purchase of this. Presume an equipment costs 100000 lakhs so your colleague can invest 50% of the capital and have a memorandum of understanding and share the equipment. Have a fixed date so that your patients are informed. By this your 50% of the capital is saved if this formula works you can go in for second newer technology and update the technologies.

LEVEL 3: Should be above 1500000

a. Space required : Above 1000 sq ft
b. Capital expenditure should be between 1000000 to 4000000
c. Again sharing of equipments can be applied as Level 2

Meeting capital needs

a. Self-financing
b. Bank loans
c. Credit card debt

d. People-to-people lending
e. Investment capital
f. Borrowing from friends

Self-financing

The owner can finance it himself or herself through savings or other available personal resources. If you are a married person you can always borrow from your wife or earning children and in return, you should pay a reward by cash or kind and return back the amount within the stipulated time. In my personnel experience I found this is the easiest way of taking loan from your family members with the same interest as the bank or more. This will give lot of confidence among the family members.

Loans

Bank Loans

The owner can also raise capital for a business using an equity loan on his home or other assets he or she may own. Many owners seek a bank loan in the name of their business, however, banks will usually insist on a personal guarantee by the business owner. Usually the bank loans are taken for equipments and the building advance. Try to earn for your day to expenditure the loan, so that you can clear the loan in less than two years. I personally feel if you're earning Rs 100000/month, 40% of your earning should go towards the loan and 60% should be to fulfil personnel needs. In this 60%, 10% should be towards the developmental fund.

Credit Card Debt

Financing a business with credit card debt is usually a poor choice; the interest rate on credit cards is often several times the rate that would be paid on a line of credit or bank loan.

People-to-people Lending

While borrowing from friends and family for business has been long-practiced, new services and markets to respond to the needs of "social finance" or "people-to-people" lending are emerging. In some cases, these online services provide a marketplace between lenders and borrowers.

Borrowing from Friends

Always a friend in need is a friend in deed. When a close friend is starting a business venture always volunteer to help financially if need requires which can be repaid at a later date.

CONCLUSION

Introduce technologies which gives faster return on investment and also it will help you to replace the older technologies.

Understanding Basic Financial Aspects

N Vishwanathan
Chartered Accountant
vishy1962@yahoo.com

4

ONE ALL-PURPOSE ILLUSTRATION

It is a case of a small tea stall. Say, our friend Soma starts a tea stall. Soma brings Rs. 1000 on his own and borrows Rs. 1000 on the condition that he will have to pay an interest of Rs. 300 at the end of every month. That's all he can borrow at present. Thus, Soma has a total of Rs. 2000, i.e. total funds available with Soma for employment in business, (accountants call it **total capital employed**) represented by Rs. 1000 of his own money (**owners' funds** same as **shareholders funds**) and Rs. 1000 of borrowed money (**debt or borrowings**).

He buys a hot plate, vessels and crockery. These are the assets he will need to make tea everyday (accountants call them **fixed assets**) for Rs. 1000. Fixed assets are assets which a businessman uses to manufacture or run his business and does not intend to sell them in the normal course of business.

Then he buys material required to make tea viz milk, sugar, tea powder (stocks or inventory, part of **working capital**) for Rs. 500. Cash left with him is Rs. 500.

On Day 1, he sells 100 cups of tea at Rs. 5 each. The tradition in the area is that you are paid on the next day. At the end of the day, Soma has not got a single penny from sales but he knows that he will get Rs. 500 tomorrow (i.e. his **receivables** or **debtors** are Rs. 500). At the end of the day, he is also left with Rs. 200 worth of stock (sugar, tea leaves etc) which is usable on the next day. **Inventory** at the end of the day is Rs. 200. He has hired a helper who would cost him Rs. 50 per day. The helper's salary will be paid on weekly basis. Besides, he has to pay Rs. 10 as interest on the loan. The amount payable to helper and interest are **payables** or more specifically **creditor for expenses**. You can imagine that in a business, you will have substantial creditors for goods also.

BASIC ACCOUNTING PRINCIPLES

Soma has not received a single penny at the end of day 1, but we know that he generated sales of Rs. 500 and material cost was only Rs. 300 (i.e. material purchase of Rs. 500, net of stock at the end of the day of Rs. 200). In other words, his gross profit was Rs. 200. We are taking into account sales and profits despite no money being actually received. This is called the **Accrual Principle**.

Consider material cost on day 1. Logically, we take material cost at Rs. 300, i.e. raw material net of stock left at the end of the day. In other words, we are trying to match the revenue of a particular period with cost of that period only. This is called the **Matching Principle**.

Imagine what will happen, if at the end of day 1, Soma has to close his business and sell all his assets. Fixed assets for which he paid Rs. 1000, may barely realize Rs. 200 in a distress sale. But in all probability, he will run his business for a long time and even if he sells he will sell as a going concern and not as vessels and crockery. So, should we take this possible loss of Rs. 800. Obviously not. The reason is that we know and we presume that Soma's business will go on, tomorrow, the day after tomorrow and later as well. This is called the **Going Concern Principle**. In other words, we presume that the business concern will continue to go on and Soma will not be compelled in distress to sell his fixed assets.

If at the end of the day, somebody promises you that he will buy your 200 cups of tea at Rs. 6 tomorrow. Will you consider that you have already made a profit? A prudent businessman will not. But on the other hand, if you discover that some of your raw material is damaged or not usable on the next day, a prudent businessman would consider that as a loss. This is called the **Principle of Conservatism**.

These are all the core principles based on which accounting is done and a balance sheet is prepared for even the largest company in the world.

Balance Sheet has to Tally

Balance sheet is a statement containing the details of where the money has come from and where it has gone. By its very definition, it has to tally. It is like saying that you left home with a 100 rupee note in your pocket, spent some money at various places and came back home. If you have lost some money, you will have to show it as a loss. All expenditures and the balance left in your pocket has to be Rs. 100 plus any receipts you might have received on the way. We will come back to balance sheet with our Soma's example.

Types of Capital

To run any business the money you raise can be your own or somebody else's. Your own money can be money received on inheritance, dowry, earned by your own hard work or as received as gift. The test that you own money is money that you do not have to account for, nor do you have to return it to anybody ever. All that is not your own money would fall under the head - borrowed money. This is the money that belongs to somebody else and will have to be returned and in most cases with some additional charge for use of that money. That charge is called interest cost.

Types of Assets

Fixed assets form the productive capacity for any business and are not traded in the course of the business. In our example, hot plate, vessels, crockery form fixed assets whereas milk, tea, sugar, receivables, payables etc form working capital. In working capital, the ones which will get converted into cash are called **current assets**. The ones that have to be paid in cash (or kind) are called **current liabilities**. **Working capital** is current assets *minus* current liabilities.

To define again, current assets are assets which are expected to be converted into cash in normal business cycle (typically less than a year) and current liabilities are liabilities expected to be paid in cash in normal business cycle (typically less than a year). Fixed assets under normal circumstances are used for a much longer period.

Depreciation

Obviously, fixed assets also deplete in value and have a life longer than one year but not eternal. So any prudent businessman would understand that he has to recover the value of fixed assets over a period of time. In case of Soma's tea business, let us say life of vessels and crockery is 100 days. Rs. 1000 worth of fixed assets will need replacement on an average after 100 days. It is as good as incurring a cost of Rs. 10 per day. Although you pay once in lump-sum, it is equivalent of paying a rental of Rs. 10 per day. When you have bought the assets the rental cost is not to be paid to anybody but it is still to be reduced on a notional basis. This notional cost is called **Depreciation**.

Trial Balance

Soma had started his business with Rs. 1000 and borrowed Rs. 1000. His activities on the first day have been discussed.

The preliminary balance sheet or statement of Soma's business (called trial balance) on day 1 will look as follows. Trial balance is a statement showing balances of sources/recipients of money. It is a combination of profit and loss account and balance sheet.

	Dr	Cr
Owner's funds		1000
Borrowed funds		1000
Sales revenue		500
Receivables	500	
Raw material stock	200	
Raw material expense	300	
Fixed assets	1000	
Cash balance	500	
Salary	50	
Interest	10	
Payable for expenses		60
Total	2560	2560

Profit and Loss Account

Soma's profit and loss account will be the same as your estimate of his profits or loss going by common sense. Let us have a look at it.

Sales revenues	500
Raw materials	–300
Salary	–50
Depreciation	–10
Interest	–10
Net profit	130

Balance Sheet

The money with which we start business will increase by the quantum of profit and decrease by the quantum of loss. Therefore in our balance sheet, the sources of total fund available at the end of any period are the funds available or

Your own money (equity)
Plus profits (if any) or
Minus losses (if any)
Plus other people's money (borrowings)
These funds are represented by
Fixed assets
Plus working capital.

Equity capital	1000
Net profit	130
Borrowings	1000
Total capital available	**2130**
Fixed assets	1000
Less depreciation	10
Net fixed assets	990
Tea/sugar stock	200
Receivables	500
Payables	-60
Cash balance	500
Total capital used	**2130**

Cash Flow and Fund Flow

For all practical purposes fund flow and cash flow are similar. In case of Soma's tea stall, the business saw a cash inflow of Rs. 1000 on account of equity, Rs. 1000 on account of debt, outflow Rs. 1000 on account of fixed assets, Rs. 500 on account of working capital and at the end of the day he was left with a balance of Rs. 500.

Cash flow statement is as simple as below:

Cash Flow Statement (Rs.)	
Source of cash	
Owners' funds	1000
Borrowed funds	1000
Total cash raised	2000
Use of cash	
Material purchased	–500
Fixed assets	1000
Cash balance	**500**

Note that in cash flow statement, we do not take sales revenue, depreciation, salary, etc. because there has been neither cash inflow nor cash outflow in the period under consideration.

We may make cash flow in a slightly different manner on the basis of activities. Working capital can be treated as a use of funds and profits as a source. This facilitated financial planning.

Cash Flow Statement	
Operating activities	
Net profit	130
Depreciation	10
Cash profits	140
Increase in working capital	–640
Net cash from operating activities	–500
Fixed assets	–1000
Net cash in investing activities	–1000
Equity funds	1000
Debt funds	1000
Net cash from financing activities	2000
Cash balance at the end of the day	500

Importance of Cash Flow

It is important to understand the critical importance of cash flow in any business. Even a profitable business can come to a grinding halt for want to cash just like a heart attack in a healthy body.

Let us go back to Soma's tea stall. Soma has no other sources of raising money. Let's presume he starts giving credit for one week, try and figure out what will happen to his business. After 1 or 2 days he will run out of cash and will have to shut down his business till he recovers his money. If he is getting credit from suppliers of milk, etc. for one day, he will not have cash to pay them on the third day!

Even if his tea business is profitable, he will not have enough money to pay his creditors and may face bankruptcy.

In case of Soma it may be still possible for him to shut down his tea stall and start his business after a few days. But in case of large businesses, the cost of shutting down the business and embarrassment can be so bad that it may be impossible for the business to restart.

Although cash flow statement and cash flow planning is as simple as adding expected receipts and subtracting expected payments. Cash flow statements are generally made on a monthly basis.

Problem arises primarily when you factor in some cash receipt which does not fructify. For instance, your receivables do not pay up in time. There will be a cascading effect. First it may affect your business and later it can affect businesses of people to whom you owe.

From the planning perspective, it is very important that one understands the probability of each cash receipt and contingency planning.

WHAT ARE DEBITS AND CREDITS?

Basically accounting requires just common sense. And given its quantity, some smart people long ago set down some rules which everyone can follow. This makes accounting mechanical and therefore one can trace mistakes easily. With computerized accounting, one hardly needs to understand debits, credits in today's world. But we discuss for the sake of completeness (love of author for the basics that he learnt in kindergarten of accounting).

In every business transaction there are two aspects:
You get or promise to get something and in return you give or promise to give something.

There is no third aspect to any transaction.

The former is your Debit and
The latter is Credit.

Look at every transaction from the perspective of the business.
Let us go back to our example

For Soma's tea stall, look at all the transactions and debit credit accounting.

- Soma brings his own Rs. 1000 into the business.
    - What business gets is
    - Cash debit
    - What business promise to give is
    - Owners' funds or Equity Credit
    - There is an underlying assumption or promise that owners will get back their money.
- Soma borrows Rs. 1000
    - What business gets
    - Cash debit
    - What business promises to give
    - Lenders (debt) credit
    - You promise to repay debt. You have to provide for interest cost also.

- Soma buys raw material worth Rs. 500
  - What business gets
  - Raw material debit
  - What business gives
  - Cash credit
- Soma buys fixed assets worth Rs. 1000
  - What business gets
  - Fixed assets debit
  - What business gives
  - Cash credit
- Soma sells 100 cups of tea for Rs. 500 on credit
  - What promise business gets
  - Receivables (Debit) debit
  - What business gives
  - Goods (Sales) credit
- Soma hires a helper at Rs. 50 per day
  - What business gets
  - Salaries (services) debit
  - What business promises to give
  - Creditors credit
  - You promise to pay salary at later date
- Raw material consumed Rs. 300
  - What business gets
  - Cost of sales (material used for earning revenue) Debit
  - What business promises to give
  - Raw material credit
- Soma hires a helper at Rs. 50 per day
  - What promise business gets
  - Salaries (services) debit
  - What business promises to give
  - Creditors credit
  - You promise to pay salary at later date
- Interest on borrowing Rs. 10
  - What business gets
  - Interest Debit (refers to use value of money)
  - What business promises to give
  - Lenders (debt) credit
  - You promise to pay interest

- For depreciation on fixed assets
  - What business gets
  - Depreciation debit (refers to gain from use of fixed assets)
  - What business promises to give
  - Lenders (debt) credit
  - You promise to pay interest

Ledger accounts refer to balances of debits and credits in each account. The debit balances get reduced by credit ones and vice versa. The net balances are tabulated in a statement, which is called Trial Balance (discussed above).

Adjustment Entries

At the end of the year, some transactions may have been missed till the time of preparing trial balance. One can pass journal entries (i.e. debit, credit that we saw above), re-calculate the ledger balances. Generally, transactions that do not take place in cash may not get left out. For instance, in case of Soma's tea stall, he had a helper costing Rs. 50 per day. He may forget to account for the same as he has not paid the salary at the end of the first day. But salary cost has been incurred and it has accrued for the business. After preparation of trial balance, you can adjust your account to give effect to the fact that profits are lower by Rs. 50 and liabilities are higher by Rs. 50. Such types of entries are called **adjustment entries**.

COST ACCOUNTANCY

Various elements of cost can be broken up in groups for better understanding and analysis. The basic breakup is in fixed and variable cost. One should not think that fixed cost always remain fixed. **Fixed costs** are costs which do not vary with volumes. In our example, tea, milk, etc. are variable costs. Because, more tea you sell, more raw material you require. But the same is not true about salary, interest and depreciation costs. Not that salaries do not increase, but it will not increase for a reasonable change in volumes. When will it change it then?

Yes, you would have guessed it. Even fixed costs static relationship with volumes is only up to a particular limit. If Soma's sales rise 10 times say to 1000 cups per day, he may need another helper and his salary cost would double. Fixed cost therefore is for a particular capacity.

Importance of Variable Cost

Contribution refers to difference of sales revenue and variable cost. For Soma, variable cost is cost of raw material. If Soma gets an order to supply tea at Rs. 3.5 per cup in a party. He should accept it provided that will not require any additional fixed asset or a new helper. And also, if supply at discounted price will not affect his regular customers.

Standard Costing

Our Soma, the tea stall owner starts setting standards.
For instance he makes 100 cups of tea from
5 liter milk @ Rs. 20 per liter (Rs. 100)
1 kg tea @ Rs. 150 per kg (Rs. 150)
2 kg sugar @ Rs. 25 per kg (Rs. 50)
He looks at the efficiency at the end of the day.
Say on day 1, when he sold 100 cups, his actual milk consumption was 4.5 liter at a price was Rs. 22 per liter. His actual milk cost was Rs. 99. Thus, he has saved Re. 1 on milk cost.

This obviously, does not give us the complete picture. He saved half a liter of milk (and therefore could have compromised on the quality) which at a standard rate would have saved him Rs. 10 (calculated at standard rate and not actual rate). This is called usage variance.

Because of higher price, he spent Rs. 9 more on the actual quantity of 4.5 liters. This is called price variance.

The saving of Re 1 consists of a high price - Rs. 10 (**Adverse price variance**) and saving of Rs. 9 on account of low usage (**Favorable usage variance**).

This sort of analysis will obviously help him plan his business better, getting better production and procurement efficiency and also in his pricing policies.

Hope, after reading this, you are in a better position to analyze Financial Statements.

Pricing

S Ravidatha
B.Com, AICWA, LIC, ICSI
Cost Accountant
ravidatha@rediffmail.com

5

Pricing of services is one of the most important as well as the critical managerial decisions which any health care organization has to make. The success of organization depends upon its pricing strategy. Pricing is one of the key components of any marketing strategy.

Many questions arise during the process of fixing the price of services. Let us look into some of these questions.

1. What is the right price?
2. What factors need to be considered while fixing the price?
3. What is the price of competing/substitute service?

Above all one needs to answer

What is the most acceptable price to our target customers?

FACTORS INFLUENCING PRICE

Profit maximization or wealth creation to shareholders is the main objective of any commercial organization. However, only this factor cannot drive the pricing strategy. One needs to consider various factors while making pricing decision. Let us briefly examine some of the important factors which have significant influence on pricing decision.

Nature of the Market

This is the most important factor which influences pricing decision of any organization. In a perfectly competitive market (where the service is already available in the market), prices are determined by market forces. In such a market, a firm is only a price taker and market is the price decider. Since, firms have limited scope in determining the prices, costs should be targeted to achieve the desired returns.

In a monopoly market or in a market where only few players exists, a firm has relatively better flexibility in determining the price of its services. For example: In India, fuel prices are determined by Government policy/objectives rather than global crude price movement. When the fuel prices were increasing rapidly in global markets, private players could not match the subsidized prices of the Public Sector Companies and were forced to stop their operations in the market.

However, one needs to be careful before taking undue advantage of such a market condition. High prices/margins will make market attractive for new players for entering into the market thereby paving way for more competition. For example, when laser systems were introduced into the medical field, similar situation was witnessed.

Nature of the Product

This is also one of the important factors for price determination. The flexibility of a firm in determining the prices depends upon factors like

- Availability of substitute or alternative products
- Seasonal nature of the product.
- Location factor of the product.
- Risk of obsolescence in terms of technology etc.
- Life cycle of the product.
- Any regulatory control on product prices. For example, Drug Controller of India, Food and Cosmetics Act, FDA etc.

Also the differentiating factor of the product when compared to its competing products in terms of quality, appearance, firm's reputation in the market also determines strength of the organization in fixing its prices. Many a times, a service commands premium pricing because of its quality of delivery and the reputation of the firm.

Cost of the Product/Service

In a monopoly or in a market where only few players exist and the product is in adequate demand, this will be the sole factor in determining the product price along with target profit. However, pricing cannot be driven solely by cost factor in a competitive market as explained earlier. In such a market, prices are determined by market forces. Again, the most challenging task would be in calculating the cost of the product. This aspect will be discussed later.

STRATEGIES FOR PRICING

Pricing is the important tool of the marketing strategy. Many a times pricing is used as key strategy to gain the market share. The intention of the Top Management should be made clear to frame an effective pricing strategy for any organization. Pricing is influenced by the objectives which a firm intents to achieve by using price as a marketing tool.

Pricing strategy is not only important for new products but also equally important for products/services which have already found its place in the market. An organization needs to continuously monitor the market developments and make suitable amendments to its pricing strategies based on market dynamics. Otherwise, there is always a risk of product/service loosing its hold on the market.

The following are some of the strategies which an organization can adopt considering the goal it needs to achieve.

1. An organization may price its services at higher levels at a premium with higher margins. This is called skimming strategy. Once the market is saturated at that price, one can reduce the prices to capture next layer of the market. This strategy is suitable where
   a. Product or Services offered is not price sensitive. This is more specifically applicable to luxury products which represent more of status symbol. For example, cosmetic procedures when initially introduced adopted this strategy.
   b. There are not too many players having significant presence in the market.
   c. The organization is in a position to differentiate its products or services from that of its competitors through quality, delivery, brand image etc.
   d. There are strong entry barriers which restrict new players (competitors) easily entering into the market. The barriers may be in the form of regulatory approvals, huge investments, low success rate, Intellectual Property Rights.
   e. The product life cycle is short and the investments need to be recovered quickly. The future is uncertain and the risk of obsolescence is very high. For example, Pager Services became obsolete with introduction of mobile services.

   This strategy has got its own merits and demerits. The main advantage of this strategy is that the organization will not be compromising on its profitability. An organization can earn higher margins during favorable market conditions. Also pricing can be adjusted during unfavorable market conditions. The adjustment may in the form of trade discounts; package offers etc. depending upon the nature of the organization.

   The risk with this strategy is that, huge margins will attract the attention of the new players into the market and pave way for competition in the market. If the new players price their products aggressively, then it will be very difficult to cut down the prices. Sometimes, this may has to be done at the cost of reputation of the firm. For example, when mobile services where introduced initially, it was priced very high. However, with the entry of new players and in spite of an increase in customer base, prices dropped drastically.
2. Another extreme strategy that can be followed is Market Penetration strategy. Essentially, this policy involves charging lower prices for services. The focus of this strategy is to gain higher market share and create strong entry barriers for new players in terms of pricing. This strategy can be suitably adopted in the following situations.

a. There are already enough competitors in the market and the product or services offered are price sensitive.
b. The organization is new to the market and wants to establish its presence though price differentiation.
c. The product life cycle is of a relatively long period and the organization can consider increasing its price after capturing sufficient market share.
d. The Investment/Fixed Cost component in the total cost is very high and profits can be improved with higher volumes through economies of scale.
e. The organization has enough resources to sacrifice its short-term profits/cash flows in order to capture higher market share.
f. The nature of the product/service is such that it can generate repetitive revenue in the form of after sales service etc. which will make overall business from the product profitable.

It can be observed that this strategy is used by many of teaching hospitals, charitable organizations, Government hospitals, new practitioners while starting their careers etc.

This strategy has its own merits and demerits. The main advantage is that it helps the firm to capture market share and customer base through its aggressive pricing strategy. It can gradually increase the prices once the services gains customer confidence in the market.

The risk with this strategy is overemphasis on market share at the cost of profitability. If the market penetration strategy is resulting in under recovery of costs, then the financial condition may deteriorate resulting in many other further problems.

METHODS OF PRICING

Cost Plus Pricing

Cost is the most important factor which influences the pricing decision. Under this approach for pricing, price is determined by adding desired profit to the cost of services. However, the crucial point is:

- What are the elements need to be included in cost of product/service?
- What amount of profit needs to be considered in price?

Cost is nothing but the resources consumed to deliver the service. All the resources utilized should be expressed in monetary terms in order to calculate the cost of product. One has to admit that, thorough understanding of the industry and organization is essential to authentically list out all the cost elements that should be considered in pricing the products/service. However, an attempt is made to explain the various cost elements that should be considered in general and also keeping the simplicity of explanation in mind.

Broadly costs can be classified under two headings.

1. *Direct Costs or Prime Costs*

   Direct costs are those cost which can be directly identified or related to products or services. This cost includes direct material cost, direct labor cost and direct expenses which can be directly related with the services.

2. *Indirect Costs or Overheads*

   Indirect costs or overheads are those cost which is incurred by the organization, but cannot be directly identifiable with the product or service. This cost includes indirect costs relating to operations, general administration expenses, selling and distribution expenses etc. In the organization is rendering multiple services, these costs need to be apportioned to each service based on some reasonable basis.

   Let us consider a dermatologist wants to start with a laser services in his practice. The following are the indicative cost elements that needs to be considered while calculating the cost of services.

Sl No.	Particulars	Cost/Service
1	Any material or consumables cost used for rendering services	
2	Direct Operator Cost (Ex : Technicians, nurses, doctors etc.)	
3	Equipment Amortization Cost	
4	Administrative Staff Cost (Receptionist, PRO, security etc.	
5	General Administration Expenses like rent, lighting, insurance, communication, printing and stationery, equipments maintenance costs/depreciation, office maintenance etc.	
6	Sales and Marketing Expenses	
7	**Total Cost**	

The above list is only indicative and actual cost elements that needs to covered depends upon the operations of the organization.

One can also classify the costs into based on the nature of the cost such as variable and fixed cost. Marginal Costing technique helps management in decision making in the midst of scarce resources as well as making optimum use of idle/spare resources through competitive pricing. However, considering the scope of the article, techniques of costing is not discussed in detail. Knowledge of Spreadsheets will be very helpful in effectively cost analysis.

Human Resources and its Importance

GN Subbanna M.com, MBA, LLB
gnsubbanna@yahoo.co.in

6

In the context of present day social and financial environment, service organizations play a pivotal role in the overall growth of economy. Service sector comprises Health, Medicare and Hospitality industry at large. World over many organizations have come into existence in the field of Health and Medicare, both in private and public sector. These organizations have nourished the idea that human resources management and development comes foremost in their agenda. Proper Counseling, Training, Team Building, Identification of leadership qualities, Motivation, Resolving conflict are some of the tools to maintain the human resources at high esteem to achieve the corporate objectives of the organization. In view of growth in life expectancy and advancement of medical sciences, providing quality services assumes greater importance and organizations have to bestow unstinted attention to development of human resources to meet the expectations of the general public.

Many organizations have taken a series of initiatives in ensuring the development of their human resources and a number of time tested systems have been put in place to sharpen the skills of employee, motivate and reorient them towards quality services. It has also helped the organizations to harness employee talent and equip them to take the responsible position in the organization to serve the patients with compassion and dedication. It is the organizations' responsibility to create greater awareness among the rank and file on the various aspects of HRD systems in services sector so that they can be put to optimal use for the betterment of both the individual and the organization. Towards this end, each organization should rethink to integrate the HRD systems in building close relationship with the internal customer, i.e. human asset of the organization. This can be achieved through effective two way communication, better interpersonal relationship, motivation and building effective career path for the employees.

In this direction, this article devotes on the following issues relating to human resources management and development:

1. Human resources development.
2. Identifying leadership qualities and team building
3. Motivation
4. Customer relationship management.

HUMAN RESOURCES DEVELOPMENT

Human resources are a very valuable asset and internal customer of the organization. Each and every employee is an ambassador and contributes to the overall business growth of the organization in his own way. It is the responsibility of the human resources managers to build a strong team and motivate the employees in all aspects to dedicate themselves to the overall growth of the organization. In this difficult task the Human resources development assumes great significance. Some of the tools available for development of human resources in service organization are discussed in detail:

Entry Interview

a. To introduce the new entrant to the history, ethos, culture, tradition and work ethics of the organization.
b. To show concern for proper induction of the new entrant and guide properly.
c. To imbibe family culture in the new entrant and draw his attention to the needs of the organization especially attending patients in the service organization.
d. To lay a firm foundation for enriching partnership between the new entrant and the organization.

Training System

a. The importance of imparting training to the employees of organization for efficient working and nurture the employee with service motto.
b. To develop the potential personality and skills of employees to perform their allotted jobs with efficiency and render good services to the patients with empathy.
c. In service industry like medicare, health and hospitality the motto should be to serve people suffering with ailments, pain, human trauma and body or skin diseases with sympathy. In training, the organization should evolve comprehensive system to sharpen the skills of employees and imbibe social culture to help the suffering people with dignity.

Incentives for Self-development

Knowledge Management of Human Resource is very essential for any service organization to face the challenges of ever advancing medical and health care industry and to march ahead in the field. As knowledge is power, constant updating of knowledge by employees is essential. Apart from well designed, established and constantly upgraded training system, organizations should pass on some incentives for the best performers to motivate others to follow. Incentives may be in the form of staff welfare measures by subsidizing canteen facilities, livery, festival gifts, arranging get-together or conducting inter-personnel competition in culture, literacy by conducting quality circle, study circle meet to bring in additional information other than medical, health care industry, for example, spiritual, banking and finance, home management, yoga etc. Moreover, the organization may also think of higher promotions to build career path and to avoid attrition or turnover of key personnel. To keep the employees with the organization, the organization should evolve all basic tenets of human resources development to keep them motivated and achieve organizational growth.

IDENTIFYING LEADERSHIP QUALITIES AND TEAM BUILDING

Leadership has often been defined as the process of social interaction and influence by which an individual or a group of people is brought to pursue a given goal and make the group to achieve the set goal.

Leadership has always been a very important agenda for an organization. Leader, captain of ship or team has to be nurtured to assume greater responsibility to lead the team and take them along with him to achieve the organizational goals. In the medical and health care industry, the Doctor or the specialist or the promoter of service industry should act as a leader and bestow personal attention to groom the people down the lane and make them to work as a team to serve the patients in unison. In medical and health care, the Doctor who leads the team of other doctors is having greater responsibility and should lead the team to greater success.

An effective leader or manager achieves their goals by organizing, staffing and properly crafting an organizational structure. Creating of jobs for accomplishing the planed requirements, staffing the jobs with qualified employees, communicating the goals to those employees and devising systems to monitor the employer's progress toward achieving those goals. Leaders try to align employees who share their vision. They create teams who understand and share their vision.

In service industry like health care and hospitals, the doctors should ensure that employees reach goals by controlling their behaviors. They should monitor results in great detail by means of reports and day to day case studies of the patients. The leader has to build a team comprising of experienced employees and others who can share their thoughts and bring out collective wisdom while delivering the services to patients with human touch. If the leader observes any lapses, non-performing or deviations from the set goals, he should conduct staff meetings and through effective communication convey his opinion/observations to build a good team. While building a responsible team, the leader should know when to praise the team members and when to reprimand them for non-performance or dereliction of duties.

The leader should also know the requisites of the team building which consists of many things such as composition of the team, how well the team is organized, culture of working together, the team's objectives and commitment, whether I am satisfied with the results, whether their needs are satisfied and whether they like my leadership in continuing with the team.

In the final analysis, as the work settings become more and more complex and involve increased numbers of inter-personal interactions, individual effort has less and less impact. In order to gain control over change, increasing efficiency and effectiveness, a team effort is required.

The creation of teams to accomplish tasks and effect desired change has become a key strategy in many organizations. Team building has become necessary as a process to control organizational change by a group whose members are joined together in pursuit of a common purpose. It needs to be emphasized here that a strong and appropriate leadership is becoming absolutely essential in order to build a cohesive team to achieve the objective set before it. The success of the team in particular, and organization in general, depends on the motivation a leader creates among the employees.

MOTIVATION

Motivation is an inner feeling, a desire and an inclination that compels a person to act or behave in a certain manner, which propels him towards personal excellence. Motivation is a feeling or a state of mind, which is specific to the individual. The only thing we can do is to create an atmosphere to build that feeling and invigorate his/her energy level to higher echelons. Motivation in the real context inherits meaning of Latin word "Movere" which means to set in motion. No movement takes place in a person until his motivation forces him to do so. An individual will remain in a state of inertia until he is motivated to do an act.

For a layman, motivation means to encourage somebody to do some work, which he is not willing to do, or not taking any interest to start the work. But at this stage, a pat on the back, a kind word, a help, a smile or an unprecedented act of benevolence may go a long way in augmenting the person's motivational instincts to higher levels and pacify him to do the work entrusted to him. Individuals are motivated by different things and in different ways. Shaping a person's behavior is like painting. One needs to use different brush strokes for different medium. What motivates one may not motivate another. For some it is the freedom that they get in their work place. For some others, it is appreciation and an assurance that their work is being recognized. For many it may be monetary benefits and for many others it may be opportunities for augmenting their learning curve. In a nut shell, motivation is simply getting somebody to carry out a task because he/she wants to do it.

Motivation is intrinsic and it is all about igniting the hidden spark in one's work life. When the leader tap into the values and desires of individuals and connect these values with the values of the organization, creativity and passion are unleashed which will help to achieve the organizational goals.

A motivated person or rather a motivated team is the secret for all successful businesses. Service Industries are not different from other manufacturing industries. The people in the service industry needs to be motivated in all possible way to serve the patients to bring back rhythm of life in them back to normalcy after such agony underwent by the patients.

CUSTOMER RELATIONSHIP MANAGEMENT

In service industry, the customers are patients or normal people who come for general medical health care consultancy, diet control, skin related matters, general medicine or counseling by the concerned consultant physician. In pursuit of service, customer relationship management assumes greater significance in understanding health of the patient, family and others who are related to the patients and take corrective steps for overall health of the family as a whole.

In Customer Relationship Management, fondly called as CRM in management techniques, relates to understanding the patients' history in total and counsel him for maintaining good health. CRM involves recording case history in detail, diagnosing the ailment, causes, family history (hereditary etc.) and remedial measures if any taken earlier and future. It also involves continuous relationship with the patients' family to know the outcome of the treatment, progress after treatment/ operation and postoperative treatment if any required. In case the ailment is hereditary, constant touch with the family members will go a long way in keeping the health of the family members under check and suggest ways and means to meet the medical requirements at any point of time. This will not only assist the family in keeping with good health of the family members but also insures against possible high expenditures at a later date.

CRM evolves around the medical history and his family members and suggest remedial measures to keep the family healthy.

In conclusion, HRM – Nerve center of an organization plays a definite role in overall development of the unit. Specially, service organizations require uninterrupted management of human resources to extend services with human touch and bring smiles on the face of the patients and their near and dear ones.

7

Ethics, Etiquette and Legal Issues

KH Sathyanarayana Rao
Consultant Dermatologist
Central Government Health Services
Bangalore
konanurrao@gmail.com

CURRENT DERMATOLOGICAL PRACTICE SCENARIO

Medical science has expanded beyond imagination, medical practice has become complicated and medical practitioners are at cross roads.[1-3] Like all doctors, dermatologists are also under tremendous pressure on various counts:

1. To earn a decent income to take care of the needs of the family.
2. To pay back the bank loans availed for financing the sky rocketing costs of medical education, postgraduation and practice set-up.
3. To face stiff competition from not only colleagues but also from specialists in other fields encroaching the field of dermatology, practitioners of alternate systems of medicine, self-styled experts and quacks.
4. To provide care for patients who are equipped with information gathered from various media including internet.
5. To counsel and convince patients with unreasonable and unrealistic expectations about the realities and uncertainties of medical treatment.
6. To prevent and face litigations from patients alleging medical negligence.
7. To equip themselves with professional indemnity insurance policies.
8. To perform in spite of administrative constraints and limitations.
9. To avoid yielding to marketing strategies of drug and medical equipment industries.
10. To remain up-to-date in the specialty by subscribing to journals and attending conferences at considerable expense.
11. To keep the interests of institution/employer/payer/insurance company/managed care organization, etc.
12. To keep academic and research interests in mind, especially in the case of those working in teaching institutions.

In the midst of all these factors, dermatologists are expected to keep the best interest of patents in mind, while providing medical care. This gives raise to ethical dilemmas[4] and conflicts[5] in day-to-day practice. Understanding ethical principles will go a long way in finding solution to such problems. In addition, being aware of rules and regulations will help to tackle litigant-prone patients and defend oneself in case of alleged medical negligence.

ETHICAL AND LEGAL ISSUES

There are two kinds of norms that the society prescribes for all professionals, more so for medical practitioners. One is ethical norm and the other legal norm. Ethical norm is a type of self-discipline expected to be followed by professionals and monitored by professional bodies; whereas legal norm is imposed by the state. When ethics fails to rein in the professionals voluntarily, the society is compelled to bring in a coercive and punitive mechanism in the form of laws and rules.

Ethical and legal issues often overlap. When they corroborate each other, there is no problem in coming to a decision. When they contradict each other, conflicts do arise and it is left to the individual to decide the path to take. But, more often than not, legal compulsions dictate the course of action. When law permits discretion, ethics helps to exercise it with fairness and justice.

OATHS, CODES, DECLARATIONS, RULES, REGULATIONS AND GUIDELINES

One has to be aware of:-

1. Hippocratic Oath
2. International Code of Medical Ethics
3. Declaration of Helsinki
4. Declaration of Geneva
5. The Indian Medical Council Act, 1956 with Amendments and the IMC Professional Conduct, Etiquette and Ethics Regulations, 2002.[6]
6. Consumer Protection Act, 1986 and Consumer Protection Rules, 1987.[7]
7. Drugs and Cosmetics Act, 1940.
8. Narcotic Drugs and Psychotropic substances Act
9. Drugs and Magic Remedies (Objectionable Advertisements) Act, 1954
10. Ethical Guidelines for Biomedical Research on Human Subjects issued by Indian Council of Medical Research, New Delhi, 2000.[8]
11. Sections 80, 88, 304 A of Indian Penal Code, 1860
12. Regulations under State Laws in r/o Medical Establishments
13. Biomedical Waste (management and handling) Rules, 1998.[9]
14. IADVL Guidelines for Dermatosurgery, 2008.[10]

ETHICAL PRINCIPLES

The word "ethics" is derived from the Greek word "ethos" which means custom or character. Study of ethics[11-15] provides us with philosophical reasoning to decide whether an action or behavior is right or wrong; good or bad. But these terms are highly relative. What is good for a particular patient in a specific situation may not be good for another patient in the same situation or the same patient in a different setting. Then, how to decide what is the correct path?

One of the approaches, called the "Four Principles" approach, developed by Tom Beauchamp, a philosopher and James Childress, a theologian, in 1970s is helpful.[16] The four principles are: autonomy, beneficence, non-maleficence and Justice.[17]

Autonomy

This principle states that the person has the right to self-determination and right to information. The positive right to autonomy allows the patient freedom to decide the course of action/treatment/procedure/surgery as well as the right to refuse treatment. The negative right to autonomy dictates that no body can force an individual to take a particular course of action. Therefore, a doctor cannot act like a dictator but only as a facilitator for the patient to come to a decision.

The right to privacy and confidentiality also flow from this principle. So, it is important to protect the privacy of the patient while examining, teaching, educating, researching or publishing and maintain confidentiality of medical data. Disclosure of personal medical information and revealing the identity can only be done with prior permission of the patient except under special circumstances like direction from a court of law, public health requirements, etc.

The concept of obtaining consent of patient for examination/test/procedure/surgery also arises from the principle of patients' autonomy.

Doctors' autonomy should provide complete freedom with respect to professional advice to patients and prescription practices. There should be no interference, pressure or coercion in this respect from any quarter.

Beneficence

This principle dictates that a doctor has to do only that which benefits the patient. All other factors have to be secondary.

Patients' welfare must be the sole consideration for starting treatment. This also imposes a duty to provide standard care for which a doctor has to be competent by possessing necessary skill and experience.

Non-maleficence

This principle, attributed to Hippocratic Oath, originated with the Roman physician Galen's dictum "Primum non nocere", which literally means "Above all do no harm". One should always ensure that benefit outweighs the risk associated with any drug or intervention advised to the patient.

Justice

This principle demands non-discrimination based on factors like sex, race, color, HIV positivity, etc. Distributive justice dictates equitable distribution of resources at macro and micro levels. In government hospitals doctors may have to act as economic gatekeepers to prioritise/ decide which patient gets expensive diagnostic procedure/therapy.

INTROSPECTION

As dermatologists we do face ethical issues in routine practice but we may not realise it.[18-20] So, we need to introspect ourselves and see whether we are:

- Practicing evidence-based dermatology?
- Obtaining a proper informed consent?
- Guilty of performing procedures for which we are not/under-trained?
- Encouraging ineffective/unproved medications/procedures and untested equipments for personal gains?[21,22]
- Medicalising non-diseases?[23,24]
- Contributing to patients' dysmorphophobia?
- Promoting/selling cosmeceuticals in our clinics?
- Using latest gadgets with little benefit but at high cost to the patient?
- Ensuring quality care?
- Criticizing our colleagues to show one-upmanship?[18]
- Neglecting patients with serious diseases/disorders by concentrating on cosmetic practice?
- Surrendering our CME/conference contents to be dictated by the industry?[25,26]
- Honest in our academic and examination related work?[27]
- Guilty of distorted and distasteful advertising?

The list is not and cannot be exhaustive. Although some issues may be tricky to solve, most of the time, common sense or our conscience shows the right path.

ETIQUETTE

Patients may not worry much whether their doctors are empathetic, but expect them to at least remain respectful and attentive.[28] It is important to develop etiquette[6, 29] – good manners – for clinical encounters, whether it is bedside or outpatient consults. Some hints are:

- Welcome with a smile or gesture, hand shake being optional.
- Offer a seat.
- Respect every patient irrespective of his/her educational/social status.
- Have eye to eye contact with the patient.
- Pay attention to patient and listen carefully.
- Do not interrupt patient's narration unless it is totally off-track.
- Be sensitive to patient's concerns regarding privacy and confidentiality.

PROFESSIONAL LIABILITY[30]

A dermatologist's professional liability falls under different categories:

1. IMC Professional Conduct, Etiquette and Ethics Regulations, 2002.
2. Civil liability to pay damages under law of torts for negligence.
3. Liability under consumer protection Act for deficiency of service.
4. Vicarious liability for negligence of assistants/subordinates.[31]
5. Criminal liability to pay fine and/or undergo imprisonment for gross negligence.

Liability under law of tort for civil wrong, depends upon the quantum of damage while under the criminal law it depends upon the degree of negligence involved.

INDIAN MEDICAL COUNCIL RULES — SOME HIGHLIGHTS[6, 32]

1. Only recognized medical degrees or such certificates/diplomas and memberships/honours which confer professional knowledge or recognizes any exemplary qualifications/achievements, should be suffixed.
2. One should not refuse to treat a patient in an emergency situation.
3. Consultation fee and other charges must be displayed in the consultation chamber/hospital.
4. It is unethical to solicit patients directly or indirectly.
5. It is improper to affix signboards in places where one does not work or reside.
6. All prescriptions should carry Registration Nos. accorded by MCI/ State Medical Council.

7. Investigations should be done judiciously and not as a routine.
8. Attending CME for 30 hours every 5 years is essential.
9. Identification mark of patient should be entered in the medical certificate and a copy of the medical certificate issued must be kept.
10. It must be a matter of pleasure and privilege to render gratuitous service to doctors and their immediate family members.
11. Unqualified assistants should not be employed.
12. A non-exhaustive list of 24 acts of omission and commission which are considered actionable misconducts, have been cited.
13. Professional incompetence is to be decided by a peer group as per MCI guidelines.
14. Clinical research/trials must conform to ICMR guidelines.
15. Complaint of professional misconduct is to be decided within 6 months.
16. Disciplinary action may include temporary or permanent cancellation of license to practise medicine.

LEGAL DUTIES TO PATIENTS[17, 30]

1. Duty of care in deciding whether to undertake the case. So, one should be competent, experienced and have essential equipments and other facilities.
2. Duty of care in deciding what treatment to give. Hence, one should have up-to-date knowledge in the specialty.
3. Duty of care in the administration of that treatment. Therefore, one should possess the necessary skill.

A breach of any of these duties gives a right of action for negligence to the patient.

INFORMED CONSENT[33-38]

Every competent adult has the right to decide what is done to his body. Consent is like giving permission. Legally, it is a contract between two or more individuals, i.e. an agreement enforceable by law. Consent will be valid only if it is voluntary and obtained after providing full information. How much information is to be given depends upon the patient and the circumstance. In general, the information expected by a prudent patient is to be given.

There are two types of consent — implied or expressed. The latter can be oral or written. Written consent is preferred as a prerequisite for surgical/cosmetic procedures. Consent form cannot have a standard format, but has to be customized. It has to be signed by the patient as well as the dermatologist.

There is no place for blanket consent. It has to be specific to:

- The person concerned– the dermatologist who has taken the consent can only perform the procedure or surgery.
- The issue/test/procedure.
- The purpose - consent given for treatment cannot be used for teaching, research, publishing, etc.

CONFIDENTIALITY[17]

As per International Code of Medical Ethics, "A doctor must preserve absolute confidentiality in all he knows about the patient even after the patient's death".

Patients are not likely to come out with personal and sensitive information unless they are sure that it will be kept confidential. Therefore, maintaining confidentiality is doctor's responsibility to protect the patients' right to privacy. We have to realise that not only paper files but even electronic data can fall into unauthorised hands. Hence, security measures have to be established and access to such data should be on "need to know basis".

MEDICAL NEGLIGENCE[17,38]

Under Indian legal system, there is no separate law either civil or criminal, to deal with medical negligence. Legally, medical negligence is the lack of reasonable care and skill, or willful negligence on the part of the doctor in r/o acceptance of a patient, history taking, examination, diagnosis, investigation and treatment—medical or surgical—resulting in injury or damage to the patient. Damage may be physical, mental or functional injury. Error in diagnosis *per se* is not negligence.

Test of Negligence[17]

The test whether there has been negligence or not is of the dermatologist with ordinary skill and not that of the highest expert. The minimum standard of skill is expected from the junior most professional also.

As per the Bolam Test,[39] the dermatologist will not be guilty of negligence if he has acted in accordance with a practice accepted as proper by a responsible professional body of dermatologists. A dermatologist cannot be held guilty if he acts in accordance with such a practice, merely because there is a body of opinion that takes a contrary view.

Accepted dermatological practice would be that which is mentioned in a standard textbook or peer-reviewed medical journal or guideline[10] issued by a professional body. Negligence cannot be directly related to the outcome of treatment as there cannot be any guarantee to cure.

Proof of Negligence[30]

Under civil law the level of proof needed is that of "preponderance of possibilities" while under criminal law it has to be "beyond reasonable doubt".[40]

It is wrong to assume negligence on the part of the doctor merely because something went wrong with the patient. The burden of proving that there was negligence rests with the patient, except when the legal doctrine of 'Res-Ipsa-Loquitor' is applicable. The complainant will have to convince the court that:

1. The Dermatologist owed duty of care
2. There was breach of that duty
3. It resulted in injury or damage
4. There was causal relation between the act of commission or omission and injury.

RES-IPSA-LOQUITOR[30]

The legal doctrine literally means "the thing speaks for itself". At a cursory look, even an average person can make out that there was negligence. In such a situation, the doctor will have to prove that he/she was not indeed negligent. Examples: Injecting Xylocaine without giving test dose, patient getting electric shock from equipment, excising a different mole, etc.

MALPRACTICE SUITS

Fortunately, very few dermatologists have faced consumer complaints.[41] Rather than medical negligence *per se*, it is the lack of proper communication with the patient that ends up in a suit.[42,43] Cases reported include – not taking/taking improper consent, improper or manipulated medical records, toxic effects of drugs, lack of expected outcome following cosmetic procedure/phototherapy/treatment for cutaneous malignancies, etc.

LEGAL DEFENSE IN CASE OF COMPLAINT UNDER CPA[30]

1. Technical defense
   a. No territorial jurisdiction
   b. No pecuniary jurisdiction
   c. Time-barred
   d. Totally free service – not a consumer
   e. Frivolous and vexatious complaint
   f. Complicated case – to be handled by civil court
2. Factual defense
   a. Suppression of material facts by patient: e.g. duration of illness, previous illness/treatment, known drug allergy, etc.
   b. Contributory negligence: patients' or attendants' action has resulted in the damage—lack of follow-up, not following instructions, self-medication, etc.
   c. Novus actus interveniens

A new act in the chain of events between the alleged act of negligence and the resultant damage. E.g. simultaneous treatment by another doctor, use of alternative system of medicine, etc.

Sec. 304 A of the IPC

Whoever causes the death of any person by a rash or negligent act not amounting to culpable homicide shall be punished by imprisonment for up to two years, or by fine, or both.

Sec. 80 of the IPC

Nothing is an offence which is done by accident or misfortune, and without any criminal intention or knowledge in the doing of a lawful act, in a lawful manner, by lawful means and with proper care and caution.

Sec. 88 of the IPC

Nothing which is not intended to cause death, is an offence by reason of any harm which it may cause, or be intended by the doer to cause, or be known by the doer to be likely to cause, to any person for whose benefit it is done in good faith, and who has given a consent, whether express or implied, to suffer that harm, or to take the risk of that harm.

Therefore, taking informed consent for procedure/surgery is a preventive step and showing that the alleged injury or damage was due to accident is a legal defense. Taking professional indemnity insurance would be a right step to cover the malpractice litigation risk.[33]

CRIMINAL LIABILITY[44, 45]

As per Supreme Court guidelines, to fix criminal liability on a doctor or surgeon, the standard of negligence required to be proved should be so high that it can be described as 'gross negligence' or 'recklessness', not merely lack of necessary care.

Unless arrest is necessary for furthering the investigation or for collecting evidence or unless the investigating officer feels satisfied that the doctor proceeded against would not make himself available to face the prosecution unless arrested, the arrest may be withheld.

These guidelines would operate till statutory rules are framed and issued by the Government in consultation with the Medical Council of India.

VICARIOUS LIABILITY[30]

It is based on the dictum "Master is accountable for the servant's deeds". A senior under whose orders a junior works, will be accountable for all actions of the latter.

Similarly a hospital or institution will be liable for the acts of its employees,[44] provided the alleged negligent act has occurred during the course of the employee's work in the said place of work.

MEDICAL RECORDS[6, 46]

Medical records must be complete, chronological, accurate and up-to-date. In-patient medical records must be preserved for 3 years. Important facts like drug allergy, taking of informed consent, advice given, procedure done, dates of follow-up, etc. must be recorded.

Unauthorized access to personal medical data must be prevented. Patient has right of access to his medical record and if requested, it must be provided within 72 hours.

CONCLUSION

A dermatologist has to manage not only men, material and money, but also take care of ethical and legal issues. Being legally right helps to avoid litigation and its consequences, being ethically right helps to have a sense of satisfaction and being right on both counts brings peace of mind.

REFERENCES

1. Pandya SK. Where is medical practice in India heading? Mens Sana Monogr [serial online] 2006 [cited 2008 Jun 22]; 4:50-61 Available from: http://www.msmonographs.org/text.asp?2006/4/1/50/27605.
2. Medical Ethics in India: A Frank Discussion between Doctors http://www.thebestmedicalcare.com/doctors/docethics.htm
3. Muula AS. Medicine and money: Friends or foe? Mens Sana Monogr 2006; 4: 78-88.
4. Pandya SK. Ethical dilemmas. J Postgrad Med [serial online] 1997 [cited 2008 Jun 22]; 43:1-3 Available from: http://www.jpgmonline.com/text.asp?1997/43/1/1/426.
5. John F. Kamp, Let's Get Real about Conflicts of Interest in Medicine, available from: http://www.awselva.co.uk/ethics.pdf.
6. Indian Medical Council (Professional Conduct, Etiquette and Ethics) Regulations, 2002, published in Gazette of India, No.14, Part III, Section 4 dated 6.4.2002.
7. The Consumer Protection Act, 1986, published in Gazette of India, Extra-ordinary, Part II Section I dated 26.12.1986 amended by Act No. 34 of 1991 and 50 of 1993.
8. http://icmr.nic.in/ethical.pdf
9. http://www.nihfw.org/ndc-nihfw/html/Legislations/BiomedicalWasteManagement.htm
10. IADVL dermatosurgery guidelines, Indian J Dermatol Venereol Leprol 2008;74: 4-77 available from: http://www.ijdvl.com/showbackIssue.asp?issn=0378-6323;year=2008;volume=74;issue=7.
11. Medical Ethics Manual, World Medical Association, Inc; 2005. p. 42-50. Available from: http://www.wma.net/.
12. Joga Rao SV. Medical Ethics, A Ready Referencer, 1st ed. Bangalore: Legalaxy Publications; 2004. p.84.
13. Snyder L, Leffler C. Ethics and Human Rights Committee, American College of Physicians. Ethics manual: fifth edition. Ann Intern Med 2005;142:563. Available at http://www.annals.org/cgi/reprint/142/7/560.pdf
14. Madhava Menon NR. Medical ethics and health care - issues and perspectives. Karnataka Med J 2000;71;2-9.
15. Francis CS. Medical ethics, 2nd ed. New Delhi: Jaypee Brothers; 2004.
16. Beauchamp TL, Childress JF. Principles of Biomedical Ethics. 5th edn. Oxford: Oxford University Press; 2001.
17. Trehan SP, Sankhari D. Medical professional, patient and the law: the institute of law and ethics in medicine. 2nd ed. Bangalore: National Law School of India University; 2002.
18. Ann Sommerville, Dual loyalties: Commentary on to talk or not to talk by Ashok Sinha, available from: http://www.issuesinmedicalethics.org/164co166.html
19. Hooyman T, Real world ethics: Maintaining harmony, promoting trust, and improving dermatology care, available from: http://www.patientcenteredpractice.com/_files/pdfs/dermatology/News_December2006.pdf
20. Praveen B E Rodrigues, Dermatology and ethics: some case studies, available form: http://www.issuesinmedicalethics.org/084lt118.html
21. Bhatt AD. Drug promotion and doctor: a relationship under change? J Postgrad Med 1993;39:120-3 available from: http://www.ijme.in/132hl060.html

22. Prescribing dietary/nutritional supplements: where is the evidence? Editorial. Bulletin on Drug and Health Information 2002; 9 (3): 65-67.
23. Moses H, et al. Collaborating with industry - choices for the academic medical center. N Engl J Med 2002;347(17):1371-75.
23. Peter Conrad. The Medicalization of Society: On the Transformation of Human Conditions into Treatable Disorders, Johns Hopkins University Press, Baltimore,2007 available from: http://content.nejm.org/cgi/content/full/358/19/2081.
24. Hadler N M, Worried Sick. A Prescription for Health in an Overtreated America, Chapel Hill, University of North Carolina Press, 2008.
25. Kagalwala TY. The conferences are a charade available from: http://bmj.bmjjournala.com/cgi/letters/322/7297/1312#14786.
26. Robert Steinbrook, Disclosure of Industry Payments to Physicians, available from: http://content.nejm.org/cgi/content/full/359/6/559.
27. Gitanjali B. Academic dishonesty in Indian medical colleges. J Postgrad Med 2004;50:281-84.
28. Michael W. Kahn. Etiquette-Based Medicine, available from: http://content.nejm.org/cgi/content/full/358/19/1988.
29. Donald Portsmouth, Professional Ethics and Etiquette available from: http://www.ethics-network.org.uk/educational-resources/a-practical-guide-to-clinical-ethics-support-2/section-d.
30. Satish M, Menon R, Rao KV. Professional accountability and patients' rights. 2 nd ed. The Institute of Law and Ethics in Medicine. Bangalore: National Law School of India University; 2002.
31. Suganthi Iyer. Hospital held liable for doctor's default, available from: http://www.expresshealthcaremgmt.com/20050430/legalities01.shtml
32. Gopinath Shenoy. Amendments to the code of medical ethics - a welcome change, available from: http://www.expresshealthcaremgmt.com/20020531/legal1.shtml
33. Rao K H S. Safer practice of dermatosurgery. Indian J Dermatol Venereol Leprol 2008; 74:75-7.
34. Satyanarayana Rao KH. Informed consent: An ethical obligation or legal compulsion? J Cutan Aesthet Surg 2008; 1:33-5.
35. Srinivas P. Consumer Protection Act and Dermatological Practice, a Dermatologists' Perspective of Medical Ethics and Consumer Protection Act: An IADVL Book. 1st ed. 2007;7-21.
36. Etchells E, Sharpe G, Walsh P, Williams JR, Singer PA. Bioethics for clinicians: 1. Consent. CMAJ 1996;155:177-80.
37. Francis CM. Autonomy and Informed Consent, Medical Ethics. 2nd ed. New Delhi: Jaypee Brothers; 2004;54-65.
38. Bastia BK, Kuruvilla A, Saralaya KM. Validity of consent - A review of statutes. Indian J Med Sci [serial online] 2005 [cited 2008 Jun 22];59:74-78 Available from: http://www.indianjmedsci.org/text.asp?2005/59/2/74/13907.
39. Bolam V. Friern Hospital Management Committee, (1957) 1 W.L.R. 582.
40. Alok Chatterjee. Should IPC Section 304A be applicable to doctors? Available from: http://www.expresshealthcaremgmt.com/20050615/legalities01.shtml
41. Sirur SP. Consumer courts. Indian J Dermatol Venereol Leprol 2004; 70:52-53.
42. Pandya SK. Doctor-patient relationship: the importance of the patient's perceptions. J Postgrad Med 2001; 47:3-7.

43. De U. Genesis and mechanics of malpractice suits - Minimizing the risks. Indian J Surg [serial online] 2004 [cited 2008 Jun 22];66:301-303 Available from: http://www.indianjsurg.com/text.asp?2004/66/5/301/13563.
44. Hariharan Nair MR. Criminal liability for medical negligence: a drastic change? Available from: http://www.issuesinmedicalethics.org/124hl126.html
45. Smreeti Prakash. A Comparative Analysis of Various Indian Legal Systems Regarding Medical Negligence: Criminal, Consumer Protection and Torts Laws, available from: http://www.legalserviceindia.com/medicolegal/mlegal.htm
46. K Mathiharan. Medical records, available from: http://www.ijme.in/122hl059.html

Health Care Waste Management

8

Compiled by:

Health Care Waste Management Cell
Dept. of Community Medicine
MS Ramaiah Medical College
Bangalore - 560 054
hcwmcell@rediffmail.com

INTRODUCTION

Health care waste is any waste generated as a by product of a health care activity. Health care waste is considered potentially hazardous. The Basel convention describes health care waste as the second most hazardous only next to radio-active waste. There are several indications which point to the hazard resulting from improper management of waste from health care settings. Thus, each and every health care setting is duty bound ethically and morally to safely manage its waste. But what about waste from veterinary clinics and research institutions which also generate substantial quantum with a greater hazard potential (especially the latter). To provide for a comprehensive and all inclusive terminology Government of India has defined that any waste that is generated during the diagnosis, treatment or immunization of human beings or animals, or in research activities pertaining thereto, or in the production of biologicals ..... at whatever name it is called so, has to be managed according to specified norms and regulations.

MAJOR ATTEMPTS IN INDIA

Supreme Court judgment dated 1st March 1996 in connection with safe disposal of hospital waste ordered that:

- All hospitals with 30 beds and above should install either their own incinerator or an equally effective alternative method before 30th November 1996.
- The incinerator or the alternative method should be installed with a necessary pollution control mechanism confirming to the standard laid down by Central Pollution Control Board (CPCB).
- Hazardous medical waste should be segregated at source or disinfected before final disposal.

Hazards due to improper Health care waste management

WHO estimates indicate that the global burden of disease annually due to unsafe injection practices is:

- 21 million hepatitis B virus (HBV) infections (32% of all new infections);
- 2 million hepatitis C virus (HCV) infections (40% of all new infections);
- 260 000 HIV infections (5% of all new infections).

Proper disposal of biomedical waste is of paramount importance because of its infectious and hazardous characteristics. Improper disposal can result in:

- Organic portion ferments and attracts fly and rodent breeding
- Injuries from sharps to all categories of health care personnel and waste handlers
- Increased risk of infections to medical, nursing and other hospital staff
- Poor infection control can lead to nosocomial infections in patients particularly HIV, Hepatitis B and Hepatitis C
- Increase in risk associated with hazardous chemicals and drugs being handled by persons handling wastes
- Poor waste management encourages unscrupulous persons to recycle disposables and disposed drugs for repacking and reselling
- Development of resistant strains of microorganisms.

THE PREMISE OF SOUND HEALTH CARE WASTE MANAGEMENT

Firstly, not all the waste generated in any health care setting is hazardous or infectious; the bulk (70 to 80%) of the waste is municipal solid waste, which is generally non-infectious and non-hazardous; 10 to 15% is infectious and 5 to 10% hazardous. If the infectious and hazardous waste is not kept segregated but is either accidentally or deliberately mixed with non-infectious and non-hazardous general municipal solid waste, the entire waste becomes infectious and hazardous.

Secondly, different types of waste need to be handled differently. Systems of segregation, appropriate disinfection/deforming/destruction needs to be set up at the point of generation of waste. There needs to be a secured method of collection, transportation and storage of waste both within and outside the health care settings.

Thirdly, safe management of health care waste is a matter of occupational safety and concern.

As health care personnel working in the STD clinics, risk of getting infected accidentally by HIV from a patient will always be there if not careful. Such risks can be avoided by following universal precautions.

Universal precautions are a set of measures taken to ensure that accidental exposure of patients and health care workers to infected blood is reduced to the minimum. Universal precautions are based on the assumption that blood is potentially infectious regardless of whether it is from a patient or health care worker, regardless of their known HIV status, and should be applied in all patients.

Tables 8.1A and B give an overview of different options available for safe management of health care waste in different health care settings.

Table 8.1A: Options for safe management of specific health care waste for a small health care setting

Sl.No.	*Items*	*Point of generation*	*Final disposal*
1.	**Contaminated plastic waste** • Plastic syringes • IV tube • Urosac bag • Vacutainers • Blood bag • Endotracheal tube • Ryle's tube	• Segregation, • Decontaminate with hypochlorite soln., (For blood bag, inject hypochlorite inside) • Disfigure.	Secured landfill, if available OR Shredding and recycling
2.	**Culture plate from microbiology lab**	Autoclave, wash, reuse/ Disposable culture plates—Autoclave and treat it as plastic waste	-
3.	**Plastic carry bag**	Treat it as general waste	Secured landfill, if available OR Shredding and recycling
4.	**Waste Sharps** • Hypodermic needles • Scalpel blade • Metal tops of vials • Broken ampoules • Vials • Glass syringe - broken	• Segregation • Decontamination/ Disinfection • Collection in puncture proof containers	Encapsulation/ Secured landfill/ concrete pit collection
5.	**Slide after smear is examined**	Disinfect, wash and Reuse	-
6.	**Glass syringe - intact**	Autoclave, reuse	-
7.	**Intact glass bottles**	Autoclave, reuse	-
8.	**Pharmaceutical wastes** • Unused vials • Unused ampoules • Unused tablets • Unused syrup	Segregation	Drugs to be incinerated/ Secured landfill; and the container treated as intact glassware or if broken, as waste sharps
9.	**Unused pressurized containers**	Release the pressure and mechanical compression	

Contd...

Table 8.1A: *Contd...*

Sl.No.	*Items*	*Point of Generation*	*Final disposal*
10.	**Anatomical waste** • Placenta • Amputated limb • Excised organs	Segregation, Collection and stored in corrosion proof washable containers	Deep burial/ transport to common treatment facility if available/ incineration
11.	**Cytotoxic waste** • Methotrexate tablets • Drugs used for treatment of leukemia	Segregation	Incineration
12.	**Radiological waste** • Radioactive iodine • Itrium 90 • Dosimeter	-	Contained and stored till its half-life is completed.
13.	**Liquid waste** • Remains of urine specimen • Blood/CSF/pleural fluid/ ascitic fluid in the lab • Remains of stool specimen in the lab	Disinfect with equal amount of hypo-chlorite solution, contact period of 2 hours	Treated as any other liquid waste.
14.	**Rubber Catheter**	Autoclave and reuse	Deep burial

Table 8.1B: Options for safe management of specific health care waste for a big hospital

Sl.No.	*Items*	*Point of generation*	*Final disposal*
1.	**Contaminated plastic waste** • Plastic syringes • IV tube • Urosac bag • Vacutainers • Blood bag • Endotracheal tube • Ryle's tube	• Segregation, • Decontaminate with hypochlorite soln., (For blood bag, inject hypochlorite inside) • Disfigure • Shredders	Secured landfill, nonchlorinated plastics can be incinerated
2.	Culture plate from microbiology lab	Autoclave, wash, reuse	If broken, treat as sharp
3.	Plastic carry bag	Treat it as general waste	Recycle
4.	**Sharp wastes** • Hypodermic needles • Scalpel blade • Metal tops of vials	• Segregation • Decontamination/ Disinfection	Encapsulation/ Secured landfill/ concrete pit

Contd...

Table 8.1B: *Contd...*

Sl.No.	*Items*	*Point of Generation*	*Final disposal*
	• Broken ampoules • Vials • Glass syringe - broken	• Collection in puncture proof containers	collection
5.	Slide after smear is examined	Disinfect, wash and reuse	If broken, treat as sharp
6.	Glass syringe - intact	Autoclave, reuse	-
7.	Intact glass bottles	Autoclave, reuse	-
8.	**Pharmaceutical wastes** • Unused vials • Unused ampoules • Unused tablets • Unused syrup	Drugs to be incinerated/ Secured landfill; and the container treated as intact glassware or if broken as waste sharps	To draft a policy for the supplier to take back the waste and treat appropriately
9.	Unused pressurised containers	Release the pressure	Depressurizing by mechanized compressor in a closed and contained room
10.	Anatomical waste • Placenta • Amputated limb • Excised organs	Segregation, Collection and stored in corrosion proof washable containers	Deep burial/ Incineration/ CTF
11.	**Cytotoxic waste** • Methotrexate tablets • Drugs used for treatment of leukemia	Segregation	Incineration/ To draft a policy for the supplier to take back the waste and treat appropriately
12.	**Radiological waste** • Radioactive iodine • Itrium 90 • Dosimeter	-	Contained and stored its half-life is completed.
13.	**Liquid waste** • Remains of urine specimen • Blood/ CSF/ Pleural fluid/ Ascitic fluid in the lab • Remains of stool specimen in the lab	Disinfect with equal amount of hypo-chlorite solution, contact period of 2 hours	Final disposal into the general sewage carriage system
14.	Rubber catheter	Autoclave and reuse	Deep burial

The final disposal options to be taken into consideration and based on this, to evolve the systems at the point of generation.

Waste management is not an issue of technologies but is everything about human attitude and behavior. Solutions for waste management need to be addressed at all the levels of hierarchy. For the technologies to be working at an optimal level it becomes vital that health care institutions evolve a human centered systems for waste management. The choices for technologies (treatment, disposal) should be made with a clear knowledge of waste streams to be managed and the goal to be achieved.

9

Continuous Medical Education

Gurcharan Singh
Prof. and Head
Dept. of Dermatology
Sri Devaraj Urs Medical College, Kolar
gsdrsingh@gmail.com

Scientific developments in medical and cosmetic dermatology continue to make it difficult for the busy practitioner to maintain their knowledge base at a level optimal to deliver safe and effective patient care. Advances in our understanding of the pathophysiology of skin diseases coupled with the introduction of new therapeutic agents in the treatment has widened the physician's knowledge gap regarding diagnostic and therapeutic approaches to skin disorders. Additionally, most dermatology practices have expanded into the field of cosmetic dermatology where recent advances in laser and non-laser technologies, newer dermal filler agents and expanded applications of Botulinum Toxin-A have challenged cosmetic dermatologists to stay current. All of these advances have led to changes in our diagnostic and therapeutic abilities, altered expectations of treatment outcomes and created safety and efficacy issues. Based on this, the need to educate the busy dermatologist is evident. Continuing Medical Education (CME) in Dermatology therefore assumes greater importance to keep abreast with latest in the speciality. Concept and essentials of any CME activity in the field of medical sciences are briefly appended below.

CME consists of any educational activity that helps to maintain, develop or increase knowledge, problem-solving, technical skills or professional performance standards so that physicians and other health professionals are in a position to provide better health care. CME includes formal courses, conferences and workshops, as well as self-directed activities such as preceptorship and directed reading.

Continuing professional development (CPD) is a term that often comes up when discussing CME. It is generally understood to cover the development of a wider range of professional skills than learning in medical subjects. Both terms CME and CPD are in use today, often synonymously. The broad aim of CME as well as CPD, however, is to equip the practitioner to perform more effectively so that the patient and the community receive optimum care.

INDEPENDENT CME VERSUS PROMOTIONAL EDUCATION

Although independent CME program and promotional education share a common goal— to improve the quality of medical care and patient health via physician's education, they employ different strategies. Unlike product based promotion, CME content is broader and more balanced and it may include discussion of off-label use of approved and unapproved products.

NEEDS ASSESSMENT

The reason for planning any CME activity should be based on good needs assessment.

Needs assessment is the systematic process of gathering information and using it to determine instructional solutions to close the gap between actual (what learners know and do) and optimal (what learner should know and do). Examples of need data include:

Expert needs: Planning Committee, Expert panels, Peer reviewed literature, Requirement of authorities (Government/Medical College).

Participant needs: Previous course evaluations, Need assessment surveys, Focus panel groups, Requests from physicians/institutions.

Observed needs: Quality assurance analysis, Epidemiological data, National and speciality guidelines, Database analyses.

Environmental scanning: Hot topics, New therapeutics, Social trends, Lay press/direct to consumer advertising.

OBJECTIVES

This should be a clear statement of anticipated result to be achieved through this educational activity. There is a hierarchial order of objectives, i.e. increased knowledge, change in physician behavior and better patient outcome.

INSTRUCTIONAL STRATEGIES

- Small group teaching and discussions
- Practicals/demonstrations
- Clinical teaching
- Lecturing.

Most popular instructional designs are:

- Lectures with Q and A 67.4%
- Case based sessions 16.3%
- Interactive hands on activities 2.2%
- Information discussion with colleagues 1%
- Least effective instructional design: lecture.

Tips for making lectures more interesting – use interactive games, use audience response system to get feedback, add simulations and demonstrations, present case studies at the end of lectures, allow sufficient time for question answers and prompt/plant questions for meaningful discussion.

To assist the learners, the lecturer should ensure that the information presented:

- Is well structured,
- Is meaningful and interesting, and
- May easily be added on to existing knowledge.

The subject matter needs to be well organized, and the organization made clear to the learners at the beginning of the presentation.

1. Three cardinal principles of lecturing are:
   - First, tell them what you are going to tell them
   - Then, tell them
   - Lastly, tell them what you have told them.
2. Clearly identify each major point: Each point when listed allows the learner to attach the details to it. Listing also indicates to the learners when a fresh point is to be dealt with.
3. Build-up a story: Building up a 'story' as the presentation progresses is helpful to the learner in many ways. It differentiates the points, showing their relative importance. New concepts can be clearly identified.

EVALUATION

It is essential that CME is evaluated in relation to improvement in the performance of the practitioner. Although assessing effectiveness of CME and its impact on practice is not as convenient as administering post-session questionnaires, CME organizers need to aim for this approach wherever feasible. If the participants are a homogenous group, a review of medical records in an institution or direct observation of practice could be considered. Epidemiological data quality assurance studies and prescribing patterns are additional parameters that would be useful as indicators of CME effectiveness.

It is important that patient care improves as a result of the CME activities undertaken by the health professionals. Therefore, when assessing the effectiveness of CME, the emphasis should be on the outcome of participation, rather than on whether the participants were satisfied with how the individual activities were organized and presented.

BIBLIOGRAPHY

1. Bennet NL, Davis DA, Easterling Jr. WE, Friedman P, Green JS, Koeppen BM, et al. Continuing medical education: A new vision of the professional development of physicians Acad Med 2000;75:1167-72.
2. British Postgraduate Medical Federation. The quality of continuing medical education for general practitioners. London: British Postgraduate Medical Federation; 1993.
3. Davis DA, Thomson MA, Oxmon MD, Haynes RB. Changing physician performance: A systemic review of the effect of continuing medical education strategies. JAMA 1995;274:700-05.
4. Davis MH, Harden, Laidlaw JM, Pitts NB, Paterson RD, Watts A, et al. Continuing education for general dental practitioners using a printed distance learning programme. Med Educ 1992;26:378-83.
5. Grant J. CME. Its validation and outcome, In: Mansfield A (Ed): CME and the Royal College of Surgeons. Abstracts of the 1st Conference held at the Royal Society of Medicine: 'British Continuing Medical Education: A Framework for the Future' (4th and 5th July). 1994.
6. Grant J, Stanton F. The effectiveness of continuing professional development: A report for the Chief Medical Officer's review of continuing professional development in practice. Edinburgh: Association for the Study of Medical Education; 1999.
7. Hadiyano JE, Suryawati S, Danu SS, Sunartono S, Santoso B. Interactional group discussion: Results of a conrolled trial using behavioral intervention to reduce the use of injections in public health facilties. Soc Sci Med 1996;42:1177-83.
8. Kuwait Institute for Medical Specialization. CME Program. Kuwait: Kuwait Institute for Medical Specialization; 2001.
9. Tu K, Davis D. Can we alter physician behavior by educational methods? Lessons learned from studies of the management of hypertension. J Cont Educ Health Prof 2002;22:11-22.

Evidence Based Dermatology

10

AL Shyam Prasad
Professor of Dermatology
MS Ramaiah Teaching Hospital
Bangalore
Prashyam2@yahoo.co.in

Readers may well ask why an article on evidence based medicine (EBM) has been included in a book on management principles. The simplest answer is this: If health care is considered as a service industry (as is increasingly the norm), and not as a noble self-sacrificing profession, (as was the perception earlier) then patients are equal to customers. They will demand service and question the rationale of treatment, and expect results. If doctors don't deliver as per their expectations, they will simply move to the next available one. However, much this may be unpalatable to doctors it is a fact of life which the medical profession needs to accept, in this day and age, as medicine gets increasingly commercialized. So, in what ways can efficient service be delivered, and the customers kept happy? In my view, if a doctor is able to convince patients that she is attempting to give them the best available treatment, half the battle is won. In this, two components are important: (a) communication, (b) proper treatment. It is the second aspect in which EBM plays an important role. Learning to practice by standards of EBM will not only make a doctor more competent, it will also ensure that she or he is more protected against accusations of improper treatment by patients or their relatives. (It can also be important for areas like diagnosis, prognosis, avoiding harm to the patient and health economics as well). Thus knowing and practicing EBM is as necessary for a doctor as managing finances or being aware of legal or regulatory issues.

A HYPOTHETICAL SITUATION

A junior resident asks a senior dermatologist which modality of treatment he would use for a six years old child with patches of vitiligo of recent onset, about ten in number. The senior dermatologist answers that in his experience, oral mini pulse (OMP) with steroids is a good option to stop appearance of fresh patches while topical tacrolimus 0.03% would be useful in inducing repigmentation. Being of a sceptical nature, the resident does not accept this at face value, and asks another faculty member, who answers "Why don't you use evidence based medicine to find out"? Not having been exposed to this concept, the resident wants to know how she could do this.

WHAT IS EVIDENCE BASED MEDICINE?

Evidence based medicine is the process of systematically finding, appraising and using contemporaneous research findings as the basis for clinical decisions.[1] The term was first used at the McMaster Medical School in Canada, where it was initially developed as a clinical learning strategy.

The four steps[1] in practicing evidence based medicine are:

a. Turning the clinical problem into a question for which an answer can be sought.
b. Making a relevant clinical search.
c. Evaluating the evidence derived from the search for its validity and usefulness.
d. Implementing these findings into the clinical situation.

THE CLINICAL SITUATION REVISITED IN EBM TERMS

Formulating the Question

Let us now go back to the hypothetical situation faced by our resident, referred to earlier. To convert the clinical situation into questions which can be answered is the first step in EBM. Possible questions which could be put are:

a. What is the best treatment for active vitiligo in a child?
b. What is the risk-benefit ratio of oral steroids in vitiligo in children?
c. Has tacrolimus been found to induce repigmentation in vitiligo?

The first of these is a general question, the second is specific question relating to harm and the third specifically requests an opinion on a newer treatment modality. These are just representative of various questions which could be framed around this clinical situation. In general, specific questions such as 2 and 3 are better for EBM purposes.

Searching for Evidence

The next step in EBM is searching for an answer to the question. For this, what must the resident do? The easiest sources of information are textbooks, but the problem with them is that they generally become outdated very fast. Some textbooks,[2] now come with electronic updates available while buying the book, and these are quite useful. An easy source of information now is the internet, but the problem would be how to prune the enormous amount of information available into something manageable, as well as ensure its reliability. An increasingly important source for answers to clinical situations such as these is the Cochrane Collaboration.[3] As part of this collaboration, there is the Cochrane Library,[4] which is a database of systematic reviews having direct answers to questions of clinical significance. A panel of experts would have searched the relevant literature for studies pertaining to the question under review, analysed the validity and reliability of the studies, and made a recommendation. The Cochrane library is thus an enormously useful utility, and can give a rapid answer to questions, without having to do detailed search or analysis. There are other sources similar to this such as the ACP Journal Club[5] or the Evidence Based Medicine.[6] The Cochrane Skin Group (CSG),[7] is one of the fifty collaborative review groups making up the Cochrane collaboration, and has already published many systematic reviews on dermatology related topics. Cochrane library offers free recommendations, although the full text of the reviews requires subscription. If these secondary sources do not give an answer to the question, the other option would be to conduct a search of medical literature directly using medline,[8] or similar tools. Medline can be accessed free of cost through the National Library of Medicine website (pubmed)[9] or through other sites like Medscape,[10] which require only a registration. Unfortunately, full text of many articles may not be available free of cost. To effectively use Medline, some basic knowledge of search engines and limits is required, which can be acquired through trial and error, the discussion of which is beyond the scope of this article.

For analysis of the data, it would be appropriate at this stage if we talked about levels of evidence.

Evaluating the Evidence—Levels of Evidence

In EBM, cognisance is placed in terms of validity and reliability on a pyramid of research studies, at the apex of which is the randomized controlled trials (RCTs), and at the base of which are anecdotal reports. The best level of evidence is considered to be from systematic reviews, which collate and analyse many studies, especially RCTs using quantitative research tools called meta-analyses. Cohort studies, case control studies, cross-sectional studies, case series and case reports follow in that order, and the least impressive evidence is anecdotal reports.

The details of these different research study designs are again beyond the scope of this article, and the interested reader is referred to other sources.[11]

The hierarchy of evidence presented here suggests that if our resident could find systematic reviews supporting the use of OMP in vitiligo, with little evidence of harm, then she can confidently go ahead and apply them to the clinical situation. If, however, the evidence is not convincing enough (e.g. not enough RCTs, or a few stray studies of insufficient vigor), then she would have to be more circumspect. It may be emphasized here that the hierarchy presented here is not absolute. For example, observational studies (e.g. cross-sectional studies) may be the best for detecting harm from various therapies is concerned. The hierarchy also makes it clear that there is no such thing as no evidence. There may be extremely weak evidence, e.g. the unsystematic observation of a single clinician but there is always evidence.[12]

Another source for finding evidence, especially for broader questions (such as the first one in our resident's hypothetical clinical situation) are clinical practice guidelines for example, IJDVL has recently published guidelines on dermatosurgery,[13] while IADVL had constituted an expert committee which published guidelines on Stevens-Johnson syndrome/ toxic epidermal necrolysis.[14] The problem with most guidelines is the fact that they are methodologically weak.[12] However, with increasing access to electronic database and exposure to EBM, at all levels, this is improving dramatically, and subjective bias is reducing. Books are also now being published, with EBM being used for treatment recommendations; one of these[15] also has a website which updates knowledge on newer trials.

Applying the Evidence to the Clinical Situation

Having evaluated the evidence, our resident must now decide on whether it can be applied to this clinical situation. Particularizing the evidence to a single patient has its own hazards, and there are some pit falls which need to be avoided. For example our resident may find no worthwhile evidence (comprising RCTs) in children for treating vitiligo, as these rarely done for them, so she may have no choice but to fall back on adult studies.

Even if higher levels of evidence are available favoring a specific type of treatment for using in an individual patient, our resident will need to consider several factors:[16]

a. Are there differences between the trial patients and this patient? – obvious ones such as age, sex, co-morbidities, or not so obvious social factors reducing compliance.
b. Are the outcomes used in the trials meaningful to this patient? Subjective improvement very frequently is a better indicator than some of the complex quantitative scales used in most clinical trials,

which may also be poorly understood by clinicians. Short-term outcomes again, should be viewed with caution, when used for chronic dermatoses.

c. Is the magnitude of benefit likely to be worthwhile to this patient?

   The risk-benefit ratio in a particular patient may be understood by use of a concept called Numbers needed to treat (NNT).[17] This refers to the number of patients one would need to treat in order to see one additional success in the new treatment, in comparison with another treatment. What constitutes a useful NNT will vary depending on the condition, personal views of the doctor and the patient. Thus, for example, if tacrolimus in vitiligo has an NNT of 100, in comparison to topical PUVA, a dermatologist would definitely question its' value, but a patient may still feel inclined to try it, if he has had no improvement with PUVA. The other part about risk-benefit ratios is that it should be understood that clinical trials may not show up rare but serious side effects, so the patient should always be counseled about this. In India especially, there is a tendency on the part of physicians to gloss over the risks of newer treatment modalities, as patients more frequently tend to believe in their doctors' judgment, and leave all such decisions to them. This can be ego-boosting, but doctors need to combine their own experience with the evidence available, and decide. It is imperative that all major risks should be explained to the patient in easily understood terms.

d. Are the patient's values and beliefs consistent with the proposed treatment?

   Many patients have their own preferences, which need to be taken into account while treating.

EXPERIENCE VS EBM?

While the utility of EBM in deciding on the best treatment option is obvious, EBM can also be implemented for diagnostic aspects including clinical decision-making and prognostic aspects. The importance of experience and clinical expertise does not diminish with the advent of EBM. In fact, a clinician should never decide on the basis of evidence alone, taken in isolation. Besides clinical expertise, which helps in making diagnoses and in deciding treatment options, compassion, sensitive listening skills and broad perspectives from the humanities and social sciences are necessary for delivering best health care.[12] All these will contextualize the patient's illness to their personalities and cultures. EBM in fact can be used at all levels-from the junior most intern to the hoary consultant. In fact, even if senior staffs are themselves unfamiliar with EBM, their willingness to admit uncertainty, to encourage skepticism and to be flexible can help a clinical team to accommodate new evidence which may contradict previous assumptions and practice.[12]

ADVANTAGES OF EBM

Besides the obvious advantage of allowing clinicians to practice rational medicine backed by research findings, EBM also has some additional advantages. It allows the development of an open mind, especially for junior clinicians, while reducing their dependence on empirical treatment options. For middle level and senior clinicians, it helps to keep them abreast of recent knowledge and partially fulfils the role of CMEs (while improving their computer skills!). With time, EBM will be used for framing guidelines of treatment for most clinical conditions, which will make development of common approaches more universally applicable. The advent of consumer activism has made patients far more aware about their rights. As mentioned in the beginning of the article, a practitioner of EBM will definitely be able to defend his treatment decisions far more effectively in these disputes.

DISADVANTAGES OF EBM

The major disadvantage of EBM is the amount of time taken to go through all the steps of the EBM process. However, with systematic reviews increasing in number, this time factor gets mitigated, as more and more clinical questions would be answered by these, and accessing these is only one step– a "search" on the appropriate website!

Another problem with EBM is cost, especially for a practicing physician. Full access can be expensive, but for most clinicians, the few lines of recommendation of a systematic review may be sufficient, and this is generally free. Medline has quite a few full text articles available free, while abstracts would be available for most articles. Institutional affiliations for accessing e-journals are tremendously useful, e.g. the Helinet Consortium[18] of the Rajiv Gandhi University of Health Sciences, Karnataka.

SUMMARY

1. Evidence based medicine is a means of deciding on the best treatment option for a clinical situation. It can also be used to determine clinical decision-making, prognosis, harm to a patient and for health economics.
2. EBM comprises four steps: (a) framing a question; (b) making a relevant clinical search; (c) evaluation of evidence and (d) implementing the findings into the clinical situation.
3. EBM can be used by all levels of doctors, and has many advantages. Clinical experience and many societal values need to be used in conjunction with EBM in delivering the best treatment options for an individual patient.

REFERENCES

1. Rosenberg W, Donald A. Evidence based medicine: An approach to a clinical problem. BMJ 1995;310:1122-26.
2. Bolognia JL, Torizzo Jl, Rapini RP. Dermatology: Text with continually updated online reference. Mosby 2003.
3. www.cochrane.org
4. www3.interscience.wiley.com
5. www.acpjc.org
6. www.ebm.bmj.com
7. www.csg.cochrane.org
8. www.medline.cos.com
9. www.ncbi.nlm.nih.gov/pubmed
10. www.medscape.com
11. Designing clinical research. Halley SB and Cummings SR (Eds): Williams and Wilkins, 1988.
12. Guyatt GH, Haynes RB, et al. The JAMA users guides to the medical literature, XXV: Evidence-based medicine: Principles for applying the users guides to patient care. JAMA,2000;284(10):1290-96.
13. IADVL guidelines for Dermatosurgery. Ind J Dermatol Venereol, Guest ed: Venkataram M 2008;74.
14. Guidelines for SJS-TEN. Therapeutic guidelines committee, IADVL, 2006.
15. Evidence based Dermatology. Williams H (Ed): Blackwell Publishing. 2nd ed, Wiley India Pvt Ltd., 2008.
16. Williams H. Applying the evidence back to the patient. In Evidence based Dermatology, Williams H (Ed): Blackwell Publishing. 2nd ed, Wiley India Pvt Ltd. 2008;73-79.
17. Lampacis A, Sackett Dl, Roberts RS. An assessment of clinical useful measures of the consequences of treatment. New Engl J Med 1988;318:1728-33.
18. www.rguhs.ac.in/HELINET CONSORTIUM.

11

Patient Satisfaction: Why and How?

Bhanu Prakash
Associate Professor
Department of Dermatology
Vydehi Hospital
Bangalore
drbhanuprakash@rediffmail.com

"Patients don't care how much you know until they know how much you care"

—Sir William Osler

To the past generation of Doctors and Public, one entered into medical profession because it was "Secure" and very "Lucrative". Gone are the days now. Today it is overwhelmed with anxiety, broken promises, pushed to work even harder and increasing patient demand. All this has made us to think twice before they get into the medical field. Especially in the last two decades, changes have taken place that has dragged us (doctors) and hospitals into the world of legal hassles, unhealthy and unethical competition.

I will touch upon the last of the points listed above, i.e. increasing patient demand. Patients are demanding a say in every thing: from where and how to have surgeries to where and when and how to have babies. The widening gap between the service provider (Doctor) and the service receiver (Patient) has led to a dissatisfied patient. Why does this happen?

We as professionals might understand the importance of updating our professional knowledge, attend CME's, Conferences, and keep pace with the new technologies. All these are factors which are not tangible to the patient. Ultimately what and how a patient measures our competence are through other tangible measures–listening to him, promptness of services, making contact with him, his non-clinical approach to the patient, etc.

Let the message be clear: Patients select doctors and hospitals that provide services that they can see and experience rather than organizations that emphasize medical and technical services that can't be seen or judged adequately by the patient.

Under such circumstances, it would be more appropriate to address these patients as CONSUMERS", though it may be initially difficult to accept it. The word consumer is derived from the Latin word consumere which literally means one who acquires commodities or services. In the same way customer is also defined as "a person who purchases goods or services". Today the patient sees himself as a buyer of health service. When we start viewing patients as customers, we recognize patient has got certain rights and thus help to be more sensitive to quality and value in health care.

Today the hospital industry is equating itself with other service industries like hotel industry, consumable goods industry. No wonder then, hospital industry has begun to employ hotel management students in their industry.

With the third party payers—employers, insurance companies, government agencies, etc. becoming a sizeable part of patient referrals, awareness about doctors being in the net of Consumer courts, optimal health outcomes with satisfied customers is the buzzword. And among all the indicators available it is the patient satisfaction which is used as the most important indicator for assessing the health service quality determinant. It is also called by various names, e.g. Patient focused care etc. but everything revolves around the fact that the patient is supreme in medical care.

Does patient satisfaction really help you? Studies have shown a highly satisfied patient helps you in the following ways:

1. They earn customer loyalty. This leads to more customers. This also means that they don't have to spend extra on advertising as satisfied customers are the biggest advertisers for them.
2. Improved patient retention. According to the Technical Assistance Research Programs (TARPs), if you satisfy one customer, he or she tells four others. If you alienate one customer, he or she tells ten, or even more if the problem is serious. Thus, when you annoy one customer, you have to satisfy three patients just to stay even.
3. They are less vulnerable to price wars. There is sufficient evidence to prove that organizations with high customer loyalty can command a higher price without losing their profit or market share. Infact in a study report published in Voluntary Hospitals of America, nearly 70% of patients were willing to pay more money if they had to consult a quality physician of their choice.
4. Consistent profitability. It is estimated that a dissatisfied patient who leaves a practice can result in the loss of $200,000 in income over the lifetime of the practice.
5. Increased staff morale with reduced staff turnover among employees. This also leads to increased productivity among employees.
6. Reduced risk of malpractice suits. A study was done in USA where the doctors were divided into two groups. One group was those who had a case sued for malpractice at least once in their practice, and another was a group who had no malpractice cases against them. One significant factor that stood out among the second group was that they spent a little more time with the patient, speaking and cordially interacting with them than in the first group.

7. Accreditation issues. It is now universally accepted that various accreditation agencies like ISO, NABH, and JCAHO, etc. all focus on service quality issues.
8. At the end of the day all these factors can only lead to significantly increased personal and professional satisfaction to the physician.

To conclude service quality has been shown directly influence patient satisfaction that in turn improves patient retention, financial performance and productivity. It also reduces staff retention and malpractice suits.

HOW TO STRIVE FOR SERVICE EXCELLENCE

This revolves around three factors:

1. Doctor
2. Patient
3. Organization.

Let us look into what is expected by each one of them.

Doctor

Undoubtedly he has the most important role in attaining to the goal. He has twin responsibilities of giving the best professionally to the patient and also as a leader of the team or the organization, to lead the team in attaining the goal of satisfying the patient. Listed below are few tips to handle the patient so as to attain a satisfying non-complaining patient.

a. Break the ice. Be courteous, express with words of concern.
b. Listen and understand. Encourage patients to tell their story. Invite and answer their questions.
c. Inform and explain. It promotes compliance. People are less anxious when they know what's happening.
d. See the whole person. See beyond the illness to the whole person.
e. Share the responsibility. Risks and uncertainty are facts of life in medical practice. Acknowledging risks builds trust.
f. Pay undivided attention. Reduce distractions, interruptions and empathize with the patient.
g. Secure confidentiality and privacy. Watch what you say, where you say it and to whom.
h. Preserve dignity. Treat the patient with respect. Respect modesty. Your words and tone should communicate respect. Expect and encourage patient autonomy.
i. Remember the family. Families feel protective, anxious, frightened and insecure. Extend yourself, reassure inform and act as advocate.

j. Respond quickly. Keep appointments. Return calls. Apologize delays. Other's time is valuable too.

The role he needs to play as a leader in shaping the organization and his team is discussed in detail in the chapter of Human Resources.

Patient

"Liking your doctor has a lot to do with getting better"

We all have graduated from medical colleges. Most of us would have gone to our college or hospital canteens. There what we expect is speedy, friendly, tasty service. But the same if we recall an instance of having gone to a five-star hotel, we would have definitely come across services like valet parking, being escorted to the table which is set with a fine table cloth, flower vase and served in beautiful china wear vessels and finally settling your bill in a leatherette case. What does this imply? Your satisfaction hinges on the kind of expectation which you harbor at different places. In a similar way, patients expectations on a good service depends on age, gender, nature of illness, hour of the day, his attitude to his problem and probably the food, traffic jam or fight he had before coming to the doctor.

Certain generalizations can be made of what the patients expect:

1. *Availability:* Always keep up the timings. Respect the timings of the patients. Even in emergencies, they expect to be informed of the delay.
2. *Behavior:* They expect you to behave in a cordial manner. They want time to ask questions and expect you to answer them which satisfies them.
3. *Communicate:* They want you to communicate with them in their language. Avoid using medical terminologies as much as possible.
4. *Doctor:* They expect you to do a good professional work of diagnosing and treating them.
5. *Empathy:* They expect care, concern and courtesy from you and your staff.

Thus, patients are left with, to judge a doctor only by certain intangible or surrogate indicators. This is unfortunate but a reality which we have to make note of.

Here are certain tips which might help a doctor or a hospital to understand the patient and serve better:

1. Recognize that patients expect a personal relationship that shows compassion and caring.

2. Recognize the patient has got certain rights to exercise when he comes to you. Various regulatory authorities and hospitals have drawn a charter of rights of patients.
3. Make sure a patient has a good first impression of you and your set up when he comes to consult you.
4. Step into your patient's shoes; see through their eyes; hear through their ears.
5. Minimize the patient waiting time to the least possible time.
6. *Problem solving:* This is perhaps the most important among all the patient related issues. I would like to touch upon this in detail. To have accreditations to organizations like JCAHO, NABH, ISO, etc. it hinges partially on a hospital's system for handling complaints specifically.

   According to JCAHO manual,

   - A mechanism must exist for receiving complaints.
   - Patient must be informed of this mechanism and of their right to complain.
   - The organization must respond to significant complaints and take appropriate actions; Patients cannot be penalized for complaining.
   - All health care facility providers must document patient complaints and their responses to them.

   The TARP has done a survey of assessing the loss sustained by an organization to measure the financial consequence of dissatisfied customers. Let's say that 150 complaints are voiced in a year. For every complaint voiced, an additional 26 complaints are not voiced. That means there are 150 × 26 or 3900 complaints, which are not voiced in that period. Approximately, one complaint in five is serious. That means of the 3900 complaints, about 780 are serious. If 50% of the people with serious complaints go elsewhere the next time they need service that means of the 780 people with serious complaints, 390 will choose another doctor or hospital next time. If the average revenue per admission is $4000, then the organization loses potential revenue of 390 × $4000 or $1,560,000 in the next 1 year.

   It is estimated that 40% of these patients or their close family members will need hospitalization in the next 12 month period. So 40% of $1,560,000, i.e. $624,000 is the revenue loss in subsequent years as they would choose another hospital. Thus the financial implications will be too heavy for the doctor and the organization.

7. Always obtain feedback with post-visit survey cards, follow-up phone calls, a suggestion box, patient questionnaires, or a referral physician survey. This will help you to identify the shortcomings if any and further correct them so as to avoid its happening in future.

Hospital

The role of the hospital, its management and the support staff is another important factor that determines the service quality provided by the hospital. Many a time it happens that, with a competent doctor and a compliant patient, the problems persist because of the policies, work culture and attitude shown by the hospital. Traditionally, hospitals have had discrete functional services such as house-keeping, pharmacy, and the laboratory. Unfortunately, this specialization has led to more fragmentation, costly care and less than ideal customer service. For example, a study describes that during a typical three to four day stay in a large hospital, a patient may interact with 50-60 employees. Building and sustaining a service oriented organizational culture is important for the success of any organization Several changes are being seen in the management strategies with the goal of serving better and improving the service quality.

Two important strategies are being presented here:

1. The following table shows the shift that is seen strategically adopted by the hospital managements. On the left hand side are the policies practiced till 1980's. On the right hand side are the policies which are being adopted thereafter.

Key shifts in management mind set

From	*To*
Provider orientation	Customer orientation
Tolerance	Higher standards
Directing	Empowering
Employee as expendable resource	as customer
Reactive	Proactive
Tradition and safety	Experimentation and risk
Busy-ness	Results
Turf protection	Team work across lines
"We-They" thinking	Organization perspective
Cynicism	Optimism

2. The second significant shift that is being seen is the change in the organizational structure. Traditionally organizations have always been

structured in a hierarchy where the management takes the topmost priority. In the recent structures proposed (Top sided) structure, the customers are placed at the top of the hierarchy and the management at the bottom.

Generally the following features characterize a healthy organization structure.

Organization culture

Clear mission and set of principles that remains consistent
Organization democracy
Autonomy and entrepreneurship
Empowerment
Open communication; shared information
Freedom to establish and negotiate boundaries
Plan for change; initiate and manage renewal and change

Leadership

Values and expectations are explicit
Collaborative decision making
Participative management
Delegation with trust
Encourage creativity and innovation
Encourage feedback
Deal with conflict without procrastination
Manage paradoxes well
Plan and set priorities and share progress
Shared vision or mindset
Tolerance for failure

Employees

Rewards explicit and clear
Maximize individual creativity and growth employee buy-in to mission feedback on performance employees feel valued, effective and in control free to take risks, to suggest

Similarly the symptoms of unhealthiness in organization can be summarized as:

Organization culture

Mistrust; "spies" report to CEO
Lack of innovation and creativity
Employees overly concerned with details and covering themselves
Criticism prevalent; readiness to file grievances
Risk-taking minimal; little initiative for new ideas
Frequent turnover of administrators
Excessive micromanagement of total organization
Communication ignores lines of authority and delegation
Managers learn of actions from subordinates

Leadership	*Employees*
Control and power centered in CEO	High employee turnover
Vindictiveness	Frequent illness
Personality driven organization, favoritism	Minimal initiative
Reward good work with more jobs	Angry outbursts
Change initiated by leader	Pessimism and resignation
CEO's actions justified as good for organization	Reluctance to change
Openly critical of employees	Passive aggressiveness
Micromanagement of line officers.	Burn-out, apathy
	Low morale.

CONCLUSION

Patient satisfaction is an attitude. Though it doesn't ensure that the patient will remain loyal to the doctor or the hospital, it is still a strong antecedent for obtaining patient loyalty.

It is an ironic fact. The better you are, the better you must be. Quality doesn't stand still. Stagnation breeds complacency and ultimately leads to death of the organization. Patient satisfaction is only an indirect or proxy indicator of the quality of hospital performance. Always look for ways to provide better patient care and soar above each and every patient's expectations. When you reach the highest level, move the bar a little higher so that you can soar that. Change is linear and never ceases. Always take time to look outside, anticipate change. Change before you have to. And create the future; do not simply react to it.

"A SATISFIED PATIENT IS A PRACTICE BUILDER"

BIBLIOGRAPHY

1. Anne-Marie Nelson, Sheryl J, Bronkesh, et al. Measuring and Improving Patient Satisfaction.
2. Department of Health, The Patient's Charter. London, HMSO 1992.
3. Eleanor C. Hein, Contemporary Leadership Behavior, Selected Readings; 5th edition; Lippincott.
4. Goodman J. Closing the service gap III. Presented at TARP 1990, Arlington Virginia National consumer survey.
5. Improving patient satisfaction now. How to earn patient and pager.
6. Joint Commission Accredit ion of Health care organizations: Accredition Manual for Hospitals. Oak Brook Terrace IL: JCAHO, 1992.
7. Lathtop JP. Restructuring Health care: The patient-focused paradigm. San Francisco: Jossey-Bliss, 1993.
8. Leebov W, Scott G. Health Care Managers in Transition: Shifting roles and changing organizations. San Francisco; Jossey-Bass, 1990.
9. Leebov W, Verghese m Scott G. Patient satisfaction: A guide to practice enhancement, Oradell NJ: Medical Economic Books, 1990.

10. Manoj Pawar. American Association of Family Physicians: Five tips for generating patient satisfaction and compliance; June 2005.
11. O'Connor, et al. Service quality revisited: Striving for a new orientation (Hospital and Health Services Administration 1995;40:4;535-52.
12. Saharkar BM. Principles of Hospital Administration and Planning, Jaypee Brothers Medical Publishers, New Delhi
13. Stephen W. Brown, Anne-Marie Nelson, et al. Patient Satisfaction Pays. Aspen, 1993;
14. Syed Tabish, Patient Satisfaction; 699.
15. The new Webster's Pocket Business Dictionary, CBS Publishers; 2001;51-63.
16. The Technical Assistance Research Project, Patient Survey.1986.
17. Voluntary Hospitals of America, Special report: Quality care, Market Monitors 1988;11.
18. Wendy Leebow Ed D, Gail Soot M A. Service Quality Improvement; AHA Books, 1993.

12

Role of Computers for a Dermatologist

GR Kanthraj MD
Department of Dermatology
JSS Hospital Mysore
kanthacad@yahoo.com

ABSTRACT

Revolution in information technology and computerization has changed the working pattern in all fields. In medicine it has changed the academic, administrative and patient management. The common applications of a computer system are electronic medical record, storage of patient data, auditing, finance, online search and access of literature, store and forward of images and data from remote regions to deliver quality health care. It is useful in participation in online academic discussion groups to obtain second opinion for difficult–to–manage cases and composition and online submission of articles. This chapter focuses on basic applications of a computer system and analyzes the above advantages for a dermatologist to use in his regular clinical practice. Computer and its application are as essential as a magnifying lens for a dermatologist.

INTRODUCTION

Computer is a system that process large data and stores it. Applications of computer for a dermatology practice are being explored since the beginning of the information technology era.

MICROSOFT OPERATING SYSTEM AND ITS APPLICATIONS

It is the cardinal unit where all the operations of a system are processed. Windows (Microsoft) and Macintosh (Apple) are the operating systems developed to run a system. The most commonly used operating system is the Microsoft. It has (1) Microsoft word (2) Excel (3) Access (4) Power point (5) and (6) Outlook Express. These are various software that are designed by Microsoft to perform basic functions.

Microsoft word is the software designed to process the words for drafting. It was released in 1983.[1] In 1989, it was redesigned for Microsoft windows. The latest release is word 2007 for windows vista. The concept of word processor was introduced by Charles Simonyi, who then called it has 'Bravo' (original word processor). The Features of word are in built spell checker, auto correction of sentences, grammar, thesaurus, office assistant and other editing features. The master template arrives on the screen with a mouse click, the page outlay can provide following features:

- Composing the text
- Editing (auto correct for spelling, grammar, thesaurus)
- Paragraph format
- Font, italic, underline, bold, superscript and subscript options
- Adding figures and tables
- Designing the tables
- Drawing tools – designing simple drawing and graphics and so on

A dermatologist can compose clinical draft and store in the system.

Microsoft Excel

It is a software with built-in infinite electronic spread sheet application (excel spread sheet) featuring calculations, tabulating the data, graphic tools and tables. The language program used is visual basic applications (VBA).

Microsoft Power Point

It is a software program designed for presentation purpose. The Current version of Microsoft office power point 2007 for windows and 2008 Macintosh operating system are available. Slide format that were initially in black and white were brought in to a color format in 1987. Text, figures, tables and other illustrations can be assembled or pasted at relevant slides for presentation purpose. Audio, animation and slide transitions are programmed and can be used accordingly.

Out Look Express

It is popularly used to compose and send e-mails. Text message can be directly typed or copied over the appropriate places over the outlook express either from excel electronic sheet or Microsoft word.

APPLICATION OF COMPUTER FOR A DERMATOLOGY PRACTICE

It is broadly categorized as follows: (a) Administration, (b) Auditing, (c) Teledermatology, (d) Online search and access of dermatology literature (e) participation in online academic Groups. The applications of a computer for a dermatologist are summarized in Table 12.1.

Storing the Clinical Data

History, examination findings, treatment, investigation report and follow-up care of patients are documented and stored as Micro Soft (MS)-Word documents. Clinical, histopathological, immunofluorescence images are archived and stored in JPEG format or adobe Photoshop. Lab investigation reports and medicolegal documents can be scanned and stored in the system.

Electronic Medical Record (EMR)

Photography and computers can enhance dermatologic visit documentation and care.[2] Usage of EMR has increased in recent times. Recent survey of personal computer (PC), electronic medical record (EMR) usage,

Table 12.1: Computer applications for a dermatologist

Purpose	*Software or operating system used*
• Store patient data.	Micro-Soft word (text) Adobe Photoshop (images) Electronic medical record Or using purpose written software
• Send patient data.	Electronic mail or purpose written web application
• Auditing patient data.	Micro-soft excel spread sheet
• Patient data presentation.	Power point
• Store and forward teledermatology	E-mail or web based mail
• Search, select and access literature using online reprint request protocol	Online search engine - Google Literature data base- Pub med. and using corresponding author e-mail.
• Online discussion groups for difficult –to-manage cases	E-mail or purpose written web based mail for online discussion

and Internet accessibility among Austrian office based general practitioners and internists revealed PCs were available to 97% of responders, and among PC users, 91% used EMRs[3]. Electronic medical records (EMR) have great potential to improve safety, quality, and efficiency in medicine. However, adoption has been slow, and a key concern has been that clinicians will require more time to complete their work using EMRs.[4] This misconception has been replaced.

There are potential benefits to electronic referral in terms of speed and incorporation of patient data held on GP computer systems.[5] Personal digital assistants are lightweight computers that provide capture of images, display, store and networking features. EMR and personal digital assistants have been used in medicine for a variety of purposes, and they can improve the provision of medical care.[6]

Administration

Registration of patients, billing, discharge, reference and discharge letters and correspondence and other administrative drafts are performed.

Auditing

Finance audit, accounts and billing, expenditure related to clinic, nursing home and hospital are managed using Microsoft-excel or out look express.

Teledermatology

Store and Forward (SAF)

A dermatologist can use a computer to receive or transfer data and clinical images of a patient with the help of a general practitioner from remote geographic regions and deliver quality care. The SAF stores patient data (digital images, clinical and demographic information) sent by GP's in an electronic medium for future access by consultants in referral centers to deliver the quality health care in remote geographic regions.[7] This process is called store and forward teledermatology. The images are rapidly transferred and stored in JPEG (Joint photographers' expert group; http://www.jpeg.org) format using the Internet.[7] This approach enables diagnosis, management, and periodic assessment of skin lesions for complete follow-up care to achieve physician and patient satisfaction.

Various authors[8-11] have demonstrated the feasibility of store and forward teledermatology. Some dermatologists have a periodic rural consultation and they have to travel to these remote regions. A general practitioner at these rural areas can send in images as and when they encounter dermatology cases. Dermatologist receives the images, analyzes and delivers treatment. Follow-up visits or in case if it is difficult to deliver treatment in the first visit or if there is a need for further investigations, patients are called for Face-to-face examination. The general practitioners can periodically collect the reimbursement and send it to the dermatologist.

Various media of data transmission are Internet, Wi-Fi and Wi-Max. Digital lines called 'Integrated services digital network' (ISDN) have data carrying capacity or bandwidth from 128 kbps to 256 or 384 kbps.[12] Wi-fi and Wi-Max are super speed wireless network connections that enable high-speed transmission of the data. Wi-Fi is wireless fidelity that enables connections to mobile devices, digital camera, computers and personal digital assistants.[12] Superior to Wi-Fi is Wi-Max (world wide interoperability for micro wave access). It is a broadband wire less access technology providing super speed access at 70 mbit/s.[12] Speed of the transfer medium is important for rapid and easy retrieval of large data.

Mobile or Cellular Teledermatology

Portable devices like cellular phones[13] and personal digital assistants[14] provides inbuilt camera to capture digital images, computing, and net working features to deliver dermatology care at a distance. They provide immediate image access and direct interaction and it is possible to obtain clarification. Periodic evaluation of leg ulcers and skin images[15] using cellular phones and Personal digital assistants are practiced. Authors[13,15] have demonstrated the feasibility of this technology.

Laptops, hand held computers that are convenient to handle and offer combined features like camera, computing, and networking are called personal digital assistants.[14] Cellular phones[13, 15] and Personal digital assistants[14] allow taking good quality images and sending them to the expert from remote geographic regions via a wireless network, e.g. global system for mobiles (GSM) and universal mobile telecommunication system (UMTS). New generation cellular phones allow to take good quality images and transmit them directly to other cellular phones (via multi media messages) and computers (via e-mail or blue tooth-wireless connection) the diagnosis agreement is 82% compared to face-to-face consultation.[13] A feasibility study[13] confirmed the importance of cellular phone in telemedical wound care. Transfer of skin images using cellular phones with a diagnosis agreement of 70% is documented.[15]

Online Academic Groups

It is a web based store and forward teledermatology practice. Dermatologists can register to academic groups'. ACAD_IADVL groups (Online academic group formed by the Indian Association of Dermatology, Venereology and Leprosy to discuss patient management and share views among the members) or Telederm.org[16] and participate in online discussion forum as and when members submit their difficult-to-manage cases. At the same time one can submit difficult-to-manage cases and seek opinion from the other members. Images with history, investigation report, clinical and histopathological images are posted online and discussions are made. IADVL academic group is a web based group mail where all registered members share each other's opinion for difficult-to –manage cases. Those of the members who have not yet registered to this online academic group can register themselves and participate in online discussion or submit their cases to deliver quality care.

Obtaining Literature: Online search access — Online reprint Request (ORR) protocol

A dermatologist updates the recent advances by periodic reading and analyzing the journals to deliver the best quality of health care to his patient. With the advent of information technology, bio-medical publications are broadly categorized as (a) Open-access and (b) Non-open access literature. The Open access to the scientific literature means the removal of barriers (includes subscription) from accessing the scholarly work.[17,18] In open-access there is a lawful free access to the journal content on the Internet and is funded by means other than reader's subscription. Non-open access journals need subscription and usually require payment to access their content. Online reprint request (ORR) is a standard protocol that uses corresponding author (CA) E-mail of a non-open access journal to obtain the E-prints (PDF).[19] ORR is rapid, cost-effective and convenient.[20] Expiration of E- mail from its usage (E-mail decay[21]) among the CA and journals not providing CA e-mail in their home page or pub med are the significant problems for ORR. ORR protocol to approach non-open access literature has been proposed[22] and its feasibility has been demonstrated recently.[19] E-print (PDF) received by providing the e-mail of the requestor using postal reprint request saves time and over come this problem. Templates are prepared, stored in the system and used for various situations are represented in **Appendix 1A to C.** This process saves time in the busy schedule and avoids typing with each ORR.

A template **(Appendix 1A)** is created with Microsoft Word (Windows XP) and stored. It consists of a uniform format of subject and text message. In the subject column it includes the name of the requestor prefixed with Dr. and highest earned degree to avoid considering it has junk mail. Text included the Purpose mentioned as 'for academic work' and giving an option either to send the reprint in E-Print (PDF) format or hard copy. In ORR mentioning the purpose of RR is important and should be incorporated as it motivates for a positive response. The purpose of reprint request gives a fair idea to the author that the request is genuine and responds positively. It saves time, as there is no need to type the text with each request in the busy schedule of a dermatologist. Name of the Journal, CA, and page, Vol. of the desired article needs to be entered each time using the copy and paste option from the template. In case of message failure or e-mail decay, reprint request templates are framed separately as illustrated in **(Appendix 1B and C)** and sent to

Appendix 1A to C: Summarizes the templates stored in the system to use for the various steps to perform the online reprint request protocol.

Sub: Request for reprint - Dr. XYZ***

Appendix 1 A: Follow **(Step; 1).** ORR to CA (Corresponding author latest E-Mail is available). (Google search or Pub med search for author's latest article/institution affiliation or use the CA e-mail address in the most recent publications)

Dear Dr. PQR***
I would appreciate receiving a reprint of your article Published in ...

(Author/s, Title, Journal, Year, volume and page number)

Please send it as attached reply mail E-Print (PDF). Your Reprint will be useful for our academic work.

In case E-Print (PDF) is not available it may be sent as hard copy. ***

(Message failure / E-mail Decay) follow (Step; 2) *appendix 1b)*

Appendix 1B: ORR* to Co-Author e-mail or affiliated institution / departmental E-Mail

Dear Dr ABC, *** ....,

I performed an online reprint request and I am unable to reach Dr. PQR .... at his e-mail............Kindly convey to Dr ... PQR .... I would appreciate receiving a reprint of his article published in................ **(Author/s, Title, Journal, Year, volume and page number)**

If the reprint is available with you, it may be sent as attached reply mail E-Print (PDF). Your Reprint will be useful for our academic work.

In case E-Print (PDF) is not available it may be sent as hard copy. ***

(Message failure/E-mail Decay/Journals not providing e-mail address) *follow* (Step - 3) *appendix 1b)*

Appendix 1C: Postal RR to CA by providing requestor's e-mail

Dear Dr. *****

I received a message failure notification while performing an online Reprint request for your published article .... **(Author/s, Title, Journal, Year, volume and page number)**

Therefore I am sending you this postal Reprint request.

I would appreciate receiving a reprint of your article Published in ...

Please send it as E-Print (PDF) to my E- mail............

Your Reprint will be useful for our academic work.

In case E-Print (PDF) is not available it may be sent as hard copy. ***

Thanking you

Dr.XYZ MBBS, MD. ***

Consultant Skin Specialist

Complete Postal address

NB: *** Subject, Contact address of the requestor, option to send E-Print (PDF) or Hard copy is a Common factor for all steps of the online reprint request protocol.

***** Post card Reprint request is addressed to Professor and Head /name of the corresponding author

* ORR-Online reprint request protocol ** CA-Corresponding author

* Please provide correct (Author/s, Title, Journal, Year, volume and page number)

Co-author's e-mail, institution affiliation e-mail **or postal reprint request** providing requestor E-mail.

A search for the table of contents using appropriate key words on the topic either from Journal home page (noting the table of contents) or pub med, displays relevant articles. One can note the title and the abstract. If the article is interesting, the CA E-mail is noted. Using the mail compose option, the subject and text from the template **(Appendix 1A)** can be copied using the cut and paste option from the template window. CA E-mail, list of Co-authors, page No., Vol. and Journal title is copied to appropriate places from the journal home page window.

CA responds positively and rapidly in e-print (PDF format). Authors[19,20] have observed 77%[20] with reminders and 63%[19] without reminders. CA responded rapidly in PDF format and most of them within 2 days.[19] Average time taken using postal reprint request providing requestor e-mail is 2 and 3.5 weeks to receive e-print (PDF) and Hard copy respectively.[19] Purpose of request should be incorporated e.g. Journal club, thesis, and project work. It motivates CA to respond positively. ORR is feasible for postgraduates, dermatologist devoid of library facilities or posted in remote setting.

Online Submission of Manuscripts

Logging and registering to the specific sites and follow the instructions to author/reviewers track the manuscript online from submission to publication.

Information/Web Portal

Online search browsing for information on conference workshop/CME and other academic activities.

Web Portal of a Dermatologist Practice Set-up

Information on patient's disease, management, health education, physician care and cost facilities are displayed on the web with the fundamental objective being to minimize the counseling time. Patient can visit these sites and then consult the dermatologists for further management. This helps to triage, counsels the patient, save time for the physician and educates the patient. Dermatoses like Psoriasis, acne and hair disorders require counseling and education.

CONCLUSION

Computers are essential in the interest of patient and physicians. A dermatologist requires computer and should be well versed with the usage of basic operating system, online search and access protocol, online participation in academic groups and store and forward teledermatology practice to deliver quality care. Computers are as essential as a magnifying lens for a dermatologist in the present day practice.

REFERENCES

1. A Allen Roy. Chapter12: Microsoft in the 1980's. A history of the personal computer. The people and the technology, Allan publishing 2001;(1):12-13.
2. Scheinfeld NS, Flanigan K, Moshiyakhov M, Weinberg JM. Trends in the use of cameras and computer technology among dermatologists in New York City 2001-2002. Dermatol Surg. 2003; 29(8):822-5.
3. Rakovac I, Seereiner S, Ratz B, Habacher W, Pieber TR, Beck P. Use of personal computers, electronic medical records and availability of Internet among office based GPs and internists in Austrian province of Styria. AMIA Annu Symp Proc. 2008;6:1102.
4. Lo HG, Newmark LP, Yoon C, Volk LA, Carlson VL, Kittler AF, Lippincott M, Wang T, Bates DW. Electronic health records in specialty care. A time-motion study. J Am Med Inform Assoc. 2007 Sep-Oct; 14(5):609-15. Epub 2007 Jun 28.
5. Shaw LJ, de Berker DA. Strengths and weaknesses of electronic referral. Comparison of data content and clinical value of electronic and paper referrals in dermatology. Br J Gen Pract. 2007 Mar; 57(536):223-4.
6. Scheinfeld NS. Creating and utilizing a multimedia dermatology medical record for a PocketPC personal digital assistant. Skinmed. 2005 Jan-Feb; 4(1):33-7.
7. Eedy DJ, Wootton R. Teledermatology. A review. Br J Dermatol 2001;144:696-707.
8. Whited JD, Hall RP, Simel DL, et al. Reliability and accuracy of dermatologists' clinic – based and digital image consultations. J Am Acad Dermatol 1999; 41:693-702.
9. High WA, Houston MS, Calobrisi SD, et al. Assessment of the accuracy of low-cost store and forward teledermatology consultation. J Am Acad Dermatol 2000; 42:776-83.
10. Tucker WFG, Lewis FA. Digital imaging. A diagnostic screening tool? Int J dermatol 2005; 44: 479-481.
11. Mahendran R, Goodfield M J D, Sheehan-Dare RA. An evaluation of the role of a store -and –forward teledermatology system in skin cancer diagnosis and management. Clin Exp Dermatol 2005;30:209-14.
12. Kanthraj GR, Srinivas CR. Store and forward teledermatology. Ind J Dermatol Venerol Leprol 2007; 73:5-12.
13. Braun RP, Vecchietti JL, Thomas L, et al. Telemedical wound care using a new generation of mobile telephones. A feasibility study. Arch Dermatol 2005;141: 254-58.
14. Massone C, Lozzi GP, Wurm E, et al. Personal digital assistants in teledermatology. Br J Dermatol 2006;154:801-02.

15. Massone C, Lozzi GP, Wurm E, et al. Cellular Phones in clinical Teledermatology. Arch Dermatol 2005; 141:1319-1320.
16. Soyer HP, Hofmann-Wellenhof R, Massone C, Gabler G, Dong H, Ozdemir F, Argenziano G. telederm.org: freely available online consultations in dermatology. PLoS Med. 2005; 2(4):e87.
17. Wren JD. Open access and openly accessible. A study of scientific publications shared via the Internet. BMJ. 2005 May 14; 330(7500):1128. Epub 2005 Apr 12.
18. Mayor S. Open access could reduce cost of scientific publishing. BMJ 2004 May 8; 328(7448):1094.
19. Kanthraj GR. Online reprint requests and dermatology literature: A feasibility study. Clin Exp Dermatol. 2009 (In press).
20. Hartley J. On requesting electronic copies electronically. J Information Sci 2004; 30: 280–4.
21. Wren JD, Grissom JE, Conway T. E-mail decay rates among corresponding authors in Medline. The ability to communicate with and request materials from authors is being eroded by the expiration of e-mail addresses. EMBO Rep. 2006; 7(2):122-7.
22. Kanthraj GR. Online reprint request: Search, access, read and update. Ind J Dermatol Venereol Leprol2008; 74:537-40.

13

Meeting the Patient on the Internet

Mysore Venkat Ram
Consultant Dermatologist
Venkat Charmalaya
Bangalore
mysorevenkat@hotmail.com

SUMMARY

Web technology provides an opportunity and a valuable tool for dermatologists to showcase their facility, outlook and philosophy, standard of care, training and competence of staff in a proactive manner at minimum of cost. Having a Website provides the dermatologist an innovative and cost-effective communication tool to market and communicate to the current and future patients. This is particularly relevant in a large country like India, with a vast internet savvy young population. The main benefits of having a Website to promote practice are: accessing more patients from a wide geographical area, reducing time spent on unnecessary consultations, convenience of avoiding travel for both patient and doctor, ensuring proper follow-up where personal visits are not feasible, clarification of doubts by potential patients, particularly about aesthetic procedures by interactive correspondence, and providing photographic examples. While developing a website, several aspects such as customization of the site, design, support and maintenance, site updates, technical assistance, search engine optimization and Web usage statistics need to be considered. It is also important to understand the limitations of a web based practice. However, internet can only grow more as a tool for marketing and web based practice can only continue to increase as more and more patients access the Web for information and more information and sites become available. In our practice, we have effectively used web technology to great advantage and describe the details in this article.

INTRODUCTION

The Internet has had a huge and significant impact on our society with in a short span of time. It has brought the world closer, together and has rendered access to information far easier than at any time before. It has brought equality in the areas of information access and also spread of information to both doctors and patients. It has cut a cross barriers of time and distance, and in a large country such as India, with a large population, wide geographical area, and limited resources, internet has been a boon. The Internet offers both a challenge and an opportunity. It offers unlimited opportunities for hospitals and doctors in India to showcase their facilities and talents across the entire globe, which would have been otherwise difficult. Rapid spread of IT capabilities has also meant a huge computer savvy population in India, which can enable us to take advantage of the technology. In the field of medical education, students can now access information very easily. Finally, our patients are now medically educated and can learn about health and disease. Thus the Internet is making public more aware and at the same time providing new opportunities for physicians in health education. E-commerce, E-launch, E-communication, web presence, cyber dialogue, E-consultation and web based practice are some of the terms that are now applied to medical practice. In short, Internet is becoming virtual yellow pages in the 21st century.

However, the human enterprise may have just touched the surface of health-related Internet practice. The use of the Internet as a vital patient care tool is a real prospect in the next few years. A recent survey indicates that the volume of commerce on the Net has grown 300% annually. According to a survey by Cisco Systems, Net sales volume accounts for $200 billion and is doubling every 6 months. And, the search for health information is among the top three reasons people use the web. The surveys indicate that people would like to improve communication with their doctors and would like to communicate by e-mail. However, the physician community is yet to take interest in this field. It is therefore important for physicians to acquire necessary skills about this exciting new tool.

OUR EXPERIENCE

Our center for advanced dermatology was started in 2003. At the initial launch of the centre itself, the importance of website was realized and two websites: www.bangaloreskin.com (for skin diseases and skin treatments) and www.bangalorehairtransplant.com(dedicated for hair loss and hair transplantation) were started. Emphasis was put on simple patient friendly language and every medical word was explained. A FAQ section with over 40 questions was included which was updated frequently as and when feedback from patients was received. Some examples of questions in this section include "What is a graft? When will I see results?" In 2004, when liposuction was added as a new facility, a third website www.bangaloreliposuction.com was started. Special attention was paid to results section, where proper photos were included. A power point presentation of the procedure was the highlight of the website. A section "what is new?" Included all new information such as papers published and presented, conferences attended, new techniques and instruments introduced. Links to established and reputed websites were provided. Care was taken to include proper physician profile with emphasis on academic data and avoiding hype and exaggeration. The websites were frequently optimized to search engines to ensure they figured prominently on search. New features such as threadlift, pixel laser were added to the website as and when new facilities were introduced. A section "what next" was introduced which advised patients how to book dates, how to reach clinic, how to transfer advance deposit, which blood tests to perform etc. As a result, we now receive about 10-15 emails daily. Each mail is personally answered by the author and clarifications provided. The patients are encouraged to send their photos based on which assessment, possible treatments and cost are discussed. Patient is encouraged to send in their medical history and lab reports by email and also use online bank transfers to send in their advance deposits. Usually 10-15 email communications are necessary for each patient before he decides about surgery. After surgery, patients are advised to communicate by email and post their results by email only. This experience has yielded gratifying results and has helped to boost our profile. We now have patients who visit us from across the globe and this has in turn contributed to health tourism.

In the background of this experience, we now describe the basics of establishing Internet presence, the issues related to online communication with patients, the necessary utilization, promotion, and maintenance of a website.

WEBSITE

The different ways a website can help in dermatological practice are:

1. New source for patient referrals.
2. Creating physician awareness about one's expertise and services in the facility.
3. Lowering the cost of postal mails and phone calls.
4. Providing online information for education about procedures.

However for websites to be effective, several facts need to be considered:

1. Website should be simple and offer direct information; complicated medical jargon should be avoided.
2. FAQ section is very important and as many questions as possible should be answered. At our website, over 40 questions have been included in the FAQ section and these have been carefully compiled over a period of time as feedback from patients.
3. Avoid hype; internet medicine is often unrealistically hyped, and though such efforts may yield short term results. In the long run, they are counterproductive.

4. Results section: A patient will be impressed by seeing results in patients; so, always include high quality results photographs. However patient's privacy should always be kept in mind while including photos. It is the author's personal belief that video of surgery should be avoided as it may scare many patients.
5. Physician profile: It is always advisable to be truthful and factual. Today's patient is intelligent and demands information which is correct. The author can cite the example of a patient who sought information from The Royal college of Pathology, UK to verify whether the author indeed was a Royal college member!

Website Optimization

Once the website has been designed, effort should be made such that the website is easily accessible on search engines- referred to as search engine optimization. It is also possible to buy special access on search engines so that the site appears prominently. These usually need assistance of a web designer though it can be done by the doctor himself.

Email Communication

Emails can be used in the following ways:

1. To establish initial contact between the patient and the doctor
2. To provide initial information and provide clarifications for doubts and questions
3. Assesment of the problem: Certain aesthetic problems such as baldness, wrinkles, acne scars, even deposits of fat for liposuction can all be assessed adequately on jpeg images sent by email. However specific instructions as to which views to be sent are important.
4. Estimate of cost of treatment: this is the most important information sought by the patient. In cases of baldness, since the cost is usually charged per graft, and the number of grafts needed depends totally on area of baldness, it is usually easy to asses the number of grafts needed and there by total cost. Similar applications can be made in cases of other aesthetic treatments.
5. Communication of investigation results, which can be scanned and sent.
6. Postoperative follow-up. In most aesthetic procedures, postoperative follow-up needed is minimal and there fore email communications are usually adequate. This minimizes the stay of the patient in the city and enables him to return to his home town. This is a great advantage for patients visiting from other cities and countries.

Email Marketing

Several service providers offer email marketing – i.e. Sending emails to thousands of prospective patients about information about the practitioner. These service providers usually have an email bank and offer such service at a cost. However such efforts can often be expensive, and not necessarily successful.

Memberships of Societies and Associations

Another way of getting E-publicity is by obtaining memberships in prestigious societies. These societies have websites which appear prominently on search engines and have a physician finder mechanism. E.g. American academy of cosmetic surgery membership yields access to provide information about its physician members. Such memberships also enhance physician profile and thereby provide additional value.

Publications in Print Media

Publication in professional journals, newpapers and magazines is another way of getting prominence on internet. Abstracts of all journal publications can be easily accessed on search engines and in some cases such as IJDVL, full text articles can be accessed too. Such publications not only enhance the reputation of physician and establish his credibility, but also increase visibility on the net. Most newspapers have prominent presence on internet search engines and any publication therefore appears prominently on searches. However the "internet life" of many these publications are short and therefore lose their prominence quickly.

Blogs and Forums

Blogs and forums offer an interactive mechanism for patients and are widely used. Patients discuss freely, about all aspects of treatment, side effects, and even physician profile. The author has an experience wherein a patient actually sought opinion about the author and his reputation on a blog, which was answered by a former patient positively and only then the patient sought surgery.

Health Tourism and Internet Marketing

Internet has greatly contributed to health tourism in India. Health tourism is a term used very often these days and represents patients arriving from different countries in India for health care. The costs of surgery and other aesthetic procedures are only a fraction of what they are in the Western countries and since these procedures are not covered by health insurance in most countries, patients need to pay for the treatments themselves. They are, therefore looking for cheaper, but safer options and internet is a great source of information. Venkat charmalaya, like many other countries routinely receives enquiries from patients around in the world. Also, a large number of nonresident Indians reside around the world and they look to treatment facilities in India, both because of lower cost and high reputation of Indian doctors.

Much of the attention in the media so far has been on cardiac health tourism. However aesthetic treatments are an important area of health tourism as our experience has shown at venkat charmalaya. Patients from across the globe have visited us, after visiting our website and further email communication. One patient visited Bangalore for a jaw surgery on Tuesday, liposuction on Thursday and hair transplantation on Saturday! This is an example of internet contributing to E commerce in health care.

LIMITATIONS OF E PRACTICE

However some limitations of this approach should be kept in mind:

a. Security: Patients may have reservations of providing photos by email, particularly women.
b. Estimates of cost are usually approximate and this should be made clear to the patients.
c. Photos may not exactly depict the precise clinical picture and hence precise treatment delivered may often change during personal examination. This is perhaps true in cases of acne scars where in depth of scar is difficult to assess on photos.
d. Legality of such consultations is always a debated issue and a disclaimer about this fact should always be inserted while offering email consultations.
e. Disnourable and flippant consultations: often emails received may not be serious enquiries and may be causual; such consultations may lead to loss of practice time. Often patients may use internet to cross-check opinion given another doctor. The author has received emails asking for opinion as to whether opinion offered by another doctor is correct. Medical ethics demand that such attempts should be discouraged.

Limitations of Website and Internet

The Internet is largely unregulated. And hence a website can also be used by disgruntled patients for causing harm too. A dissatisfied patient once threatened the author that he will write adversely in a blog unless the fee paid by him is refunded!!!

A medico-legal issue concerns the use of email, where matters of privacy, security and confidentiality in relation to medical information exist. As per guidelines of The American Medical Informatics Association (http://www.amia.org/), the following need to be adhered to: (1) not using email for urgent serious matters, (2) informing patients about who actually handles the received messages, (3) establishing the types of transactions permitted using email, and (4) instructing patients to note the type of transaction in the subject line of the message to allow filtering.

An unacceptable offshoot of internet practice is that many patients may use email for getting opinion so as to avoid consultation fees, even if they are in a position to visit the clinic for personal examination. The author has had a number of requests from with in Bangalore for opinion. These need to be discouraged politely, but firmly.

Another area in the field in dermatology with respect to the use of internet is dermatopathology or teledermatopathology. The author being a dermatopathologist, frequently receives requests for opinion about photomicrographs sent by email. Interpretation of histological photomicrographs is fraught with difficulties particularly in inflammatory diseases. As such this area has to be approached carefully.

An offshoot of the boom in health tourism has been the development of health portals. Several health portals have sprung up, ostensibly to facilitate such patients who wish to travel for health tourism. These portals seek to assist patients in identifying doctors, arranging for travel, accommodation and treatments etc- in short claim to offer door to door service. In return they charge a fee, which is usually calculated as part of the total medical expenses. However such portals are often too aggressive marketing and do not allow direct communication between patient and doctors. As a result, the doctor is often unaware of many details about the patient leadings to misinformation. The author had an experience with a portal which offered to bring a patient of liposuction only to find that when the patient arrived for surgery, she did not need liposuction at all!

Technical Difficulties Associated with Web Based Practice

While maintaining a website is easy, and is usually trouble free, frequently difficulties may arise. Links may stop working. A web designer and provider should always be hired to maintain the sites. Websites need to be renewed promptly. The author had the experience where in the renewal of the website got delayed by a week, with resultant loss of patient communication. Considerable amount of time may be spent on answering emails, and secretarial assistance is only of limited value as may of the questions need to be answered by the physician himself. The physician needs therefore to be trained properly in the use of computer.

SUMMARY-12 WAYS TO ESTABLISH E PRESENCE

Internet is here to stay and physicians need to make the best possible use of the vast potential that this medium offers. Bill gates coined the term "health care at the speed of thought "to explain the role of internet in health care. To exploit the unlimited opportunities that this medium provides effectively, the following twelve tips are offered:

1. Identify the facility you would like to highlight on the internet.
2. Study other websites available and design a website which is user friendly, simple and has an easy flow
3. Use simple language avoiding medical jargon and clarify all medical terms
4. Showcase your photographs with high quality before and after photos
5. Avoid hype; remember the adage- it is always better to undersell and over deliver
6. Be accessible- reply to emails with in a day of their receipt.
7. Be patient; don't get irritated by the queries
8. Answer the mails your self- don't leave it entirely to your secretary- she does not have the technical knowledge that is needed to answer most questions.
9. Hire a good web engineer to service your website frequently
10. Always update the website with new information
11. Become a member of a prominent and prestigious professional association.
12. Contribute articles on professional journals and print media.

Finally, always remember: net is only a tool- it is not a replacement for conventional physician skills of proper examination and diagnosis, case selection, adequate training and enhancement of skills, and most importantly proper physician patient relationship.

BIBLIOGRAPHY

1. Arthur C. Huntley The Internet, World Wide Web, and the Practice of Dermatology. Dermatology Online Journal 2000;2(1):10.
2. Cochrane JD. Healthcare @ the speed of thought Integr Healthc Rep. 1999;1-14, 16-7.
3. D John. Doyle the Internet, Medical Practice, and Medical Education - Some Medico-Legal Issues Canadian Journal of Anesthesia 2002:49:1095-97.
4. Finch T. Marketing your medical practice with an effective web presence J Med Pract Manage. 2004;20(3):143-7.
5. Miller SA, Forrest JL. Dental practice websites. Creating a Web presence Dent Clin North Am. 2002;46(3):463-75.
6. Nagel M. Six ways to establish a Web presence J Med Pract Manage. 2000; 16(1):39-41.
7. Rothschild MA Marketing your practice on the Internet Otolaryngol Clin North Am. 2002;35(6):1149-61.
8. Toth CL, Goldstein D. Eight ways to go "e" without launching a Web service J Med Pract Manage. 2000;16(1):34-8.
9. Ullrich PF Jr, Vaccaro AR. Patient education on the internet. Opportunities and pitfalls Spine. 2002 Apr 1; 27(7):E185-8.
10. Wald HS, Dube CE, Anthony DC. Untangling the Web—the impact of Internet use on health care and the physician-patient relationship Patient Educ Couns. 2007;68(3):218-24.

14

Interprofessional Relations

S Sacchidanand
Registrar (Evaluation)
Rajiv Gandhi University of Health Sciences
Bangalore

Medicine is one of the oldest professions known to us. It is deemed to be present since the inception of mankind. The scientific evidence to our professional existence can be traced to over 2000 years back in ancient Greece. Among their works, a collection of 72 books that contain remedies of diseases and guidelines about the behavior of physicians from which the present "The Hippocratic Oath" has evolved has been traced. The hippocratic oath lays down duties, the physicians undertake toward patients as an ethical code and also lays our duties towards our professional colleagues as a covenant. Thus we can see that the duties of a doctor and his relation with other doctors are not something new.

Over a period of time medical practice has evolved as a science. Particularly in the last century or so rapid advances have taken place which has helped men to lead a more lengthier life and also has helped us to combat the menace of diseases which has been a curse to mankind.

However, it has not been all that simple as said. With the rapid rise in the advances, various features have also characterized it :

(1). Increasing number of specialties leading to specialists and super specialists among doctors. (2). Increasing number of paramedical specialists—nursing, physiotherapists, social workers, laboratory technicians, and other non medical people like front desk people, security, house keeping etc.

Thus if we look at our practice, various people with whom we need to do work collaboratively are:

1. Other medical professionals: E.g. physicians, plastic surgeons, pediatricians, immunologists etc., with whom we interact very often. In the interaction with several of these professional colleagues during the care of the patients, various levels of conflict can arise. This can lead to breakdown in communication and failure to deliver proper care to the patient. A study has shown that the lack of communication and any kind of misunderstanding may be responsible for as much as 70% of the adverse events currently reported.
2. Nursing professionals: It is important we understand here that nurses are a profession by themselves and should not be taken as people working for us.
3. Paramedical people: A few lab technicians, social workers etc. many a times think themselves to be professionals and they feel that they are the master of their specialties and they know much more than what the physician knows about that particular subject. It rests upon the physician to handle such individuals and events tactfully without offending their ego.

4. Non-allopathic doctors and healers: Qualified non-allopathic practitioners like Ayurvedic, homeopathic, Unani specialists form a big group of practitioners. In addition we have many unqualified doctors who can give various forms of medicines from various kinds of medicinal plants and food-stuff who are traditionally called as "healers." Inevitably we see a lot of patients who would have come to us after having sought the advice of these doctors or who window shop these doctors also after having been seen by us. It is important to understand the role played by these people. We have to recognize the fact that legally all these practices have been recognized as a scientific form of medical practice. It is imperative that we should desist from talking loosely about the system of medicine or the practitioners.

It has become imperative that we need to understand, live and work with these various other care takers (doctors and non doctors alike) so as to achieve the goal of optimal patient care outcome and high professional satisfaction.

In the above context it is inevitable we understand the importance of group working, the dynamics of group working. Effective inter professional working is widely considered as essential to high quality health care. This is greatly influenced by the attitudes we wear not only to ourselves, but also to other professional groups.

Broadly a group or a team is defined as when two or more persons with varied skills are associated together.

The following issues are considered important to determine the success of the team as a group, namely:

a. The individual in the group.
b. Team size.
c. Group norms, tasks, objectives, structure and accountability.
d. Democracy, to respect alternate viewpoints.
e. Decision making and conflict resolution, ability to set aside differences.
f. Communication.
g. Good Leadership.
h. Group harmony and its relationship to group productivity.
i. Trust and compromise.

Collaborative medicine requires practitioners and disciplines with varied training and philosophies to work together toward a common clinical goal. Distinct differences between the various practitioners and disciplines can serve as both opportunities for synergy and barriers to collaboration. Try to maintain the following points, which can indicate as good professional courtesies.

1. Always focus on the well-being of the patient. Refer the patients whenever, required to other professional colleagues. Don't engage the patients as your source of business.
2. Maintain an open line of communication with other professional colleagues.
3. Remember that each professional has a role to play in the well-being of the patient. A team effort will always lead to a better outcome than a fractured approach.
4. Always be careful of giving information to the patient in such a way that you are not contradicting the other professional colleague. Desist from using any patient as a medium to spread criticism of fellow professionals.

Professional Association

"Every man owes some of his time to the up building of the profession to which he belongs."

—Theodore Roosevelt

The involvement in professional association gives us an opportunity to give back to the profession for whatever it has helped us to be. It lends credibility to both the individual and also to the association. If there are any issues either of the specialty or of any interprofessional issues, it is best handled by the association. When the association is strong and powerful, it helps to provide stability within the profession as well as a strong voice when professional interests must be brought to the attention of health care policy makers. The classical example I would like to highlight was when the Indian Medical Association took up against various agencies to safeguard the interests of the doctors when the Government of India brought the legislature of Consumer Protection Act. Another example was when the Medical Council of India laid down the professional code of Ethics at the beginning of the century to ensure that the interests of the doctors and the patients are well served.

A strong association can also take up certain public awareness issues to educate the people about the common illness of public importance. A classical example is the campaign rendered by the Australian Medical and Dermatological Associations in league with various pharmaceutical companies, to educate the people regarding the importance of sun protection in the prevention of melanoma which is highly prevalent in that country.

Interprofessional relationships are strengthened when individuals make an effort to establish and maintain relationships on a personal basis and when professional associations work together to coordinate interprofessional programs and activities.

REFERENCE

Compiled from Internet sources.

Index